TENNIS BEGINS
AT TWO

A Compendium for the Surprised Parent Who Suddenly Hears, "Mommy, Daddy, will you teach me to play tennis?"

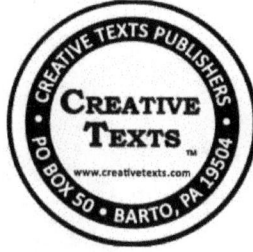

Tennis Begins At Two:
A Compendium for the Surprised Parent Who Suddenly Hears,
"Mommy, Daddy, will you teach me to play tennis?"
By Kie Foreman and Don DeNevi

Published by Creative Texts Publishers, LLC
PO Box 50
Barto, PA 19504
www.creativetexts.com
ISBN: 978-1-64738-116-5

A Word from the Authors

In the summer of 1889, the newly published textbook, "Physiological Notes on the Study of Language", Vol. XLV-49, N.Y., introduced a chapter written by Dr. Mary Putnam Jacobi.

On page 49, "Experiment in Primary Education", she wrote, "Thrice happy the child whose earliest years are prismatic with the light of the past, who lives in a golden haze through which love shines, in which all good things open, and the mind develops in even pace with a healthy play-loving body. In those years, too, often left fallow of all sowing but that of wasting weeds, how much can be done when love, and scientific training, and maternal aptitude encircle the little boy or girl?"

Abounding in energetic expressions of tennis axioms, profound yet tender maxims from champion authorities themselves, pithy old adages and current proverbs and aphorisms, this long-in-the-making cornucopia of court drama and its established principles, universally received lessons, and self-evident truths are ready for parental instruction.

Having this frontispiece greet you before your eyes read the title page, we, the co-authors, introduce you to the best ever of all tennis teachers, Helen Irene Driver, PhD. She wrote in her laudable "Tennis for Teachers", 1936, with more than 25,000 copies in over 50 countries of the World Community at that time-

"As a final please for more emphasis on social tennis and doubles play, tennis like skating, swimming, and bicycle riding - - once learned in childhood, in never forgotten. Teach the child to GET THE BALL OVER THE NET and his or her hand-eye coordination is established. Regardless of the level of his or her performance (as far as good form is concerned), the player can enjoy the game throughout life and should have no difficulty finding three others like him (or her)self to engage in doubles for fun and exercise." *

*Helen Irene Driver, Tennis for Teachers, 1st Edition, 1936, 10 editions later, enlarged edition, 1970.

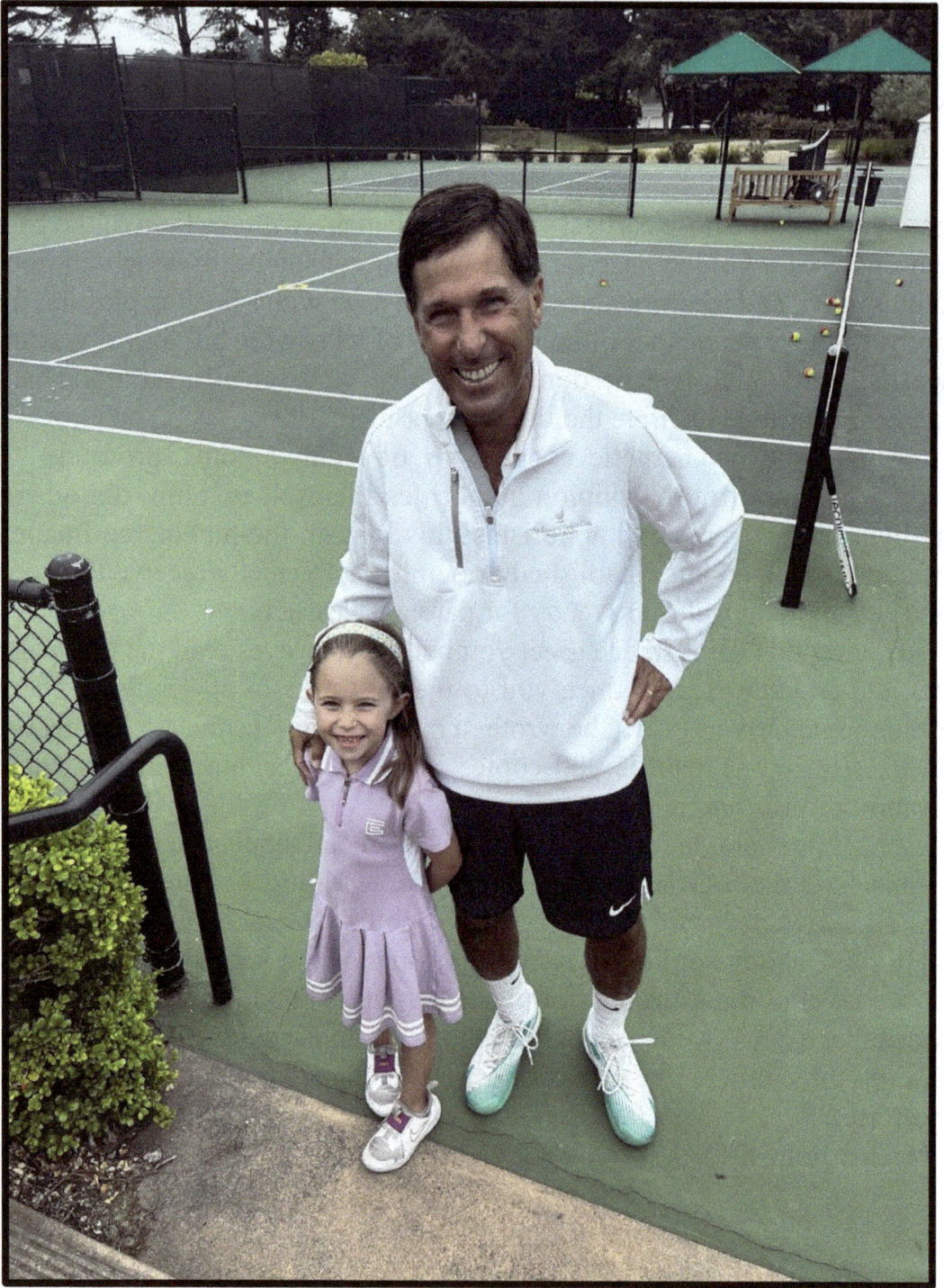

(Kie Foreman and Juliet)

TENNIS BEGINS AT TWO

A Compendium for the Surprised Parent Who Suddenly Hears,

"Mommy, Daddy, will you teach me to play tennis?"

by

Kie Foreman and Don DeNevi

Photography by David Day

Volume One of Three
Vol. 2, Ages 6 to 10
Vol.3, 11 to 21

TENNIS BEGINS AT TWO

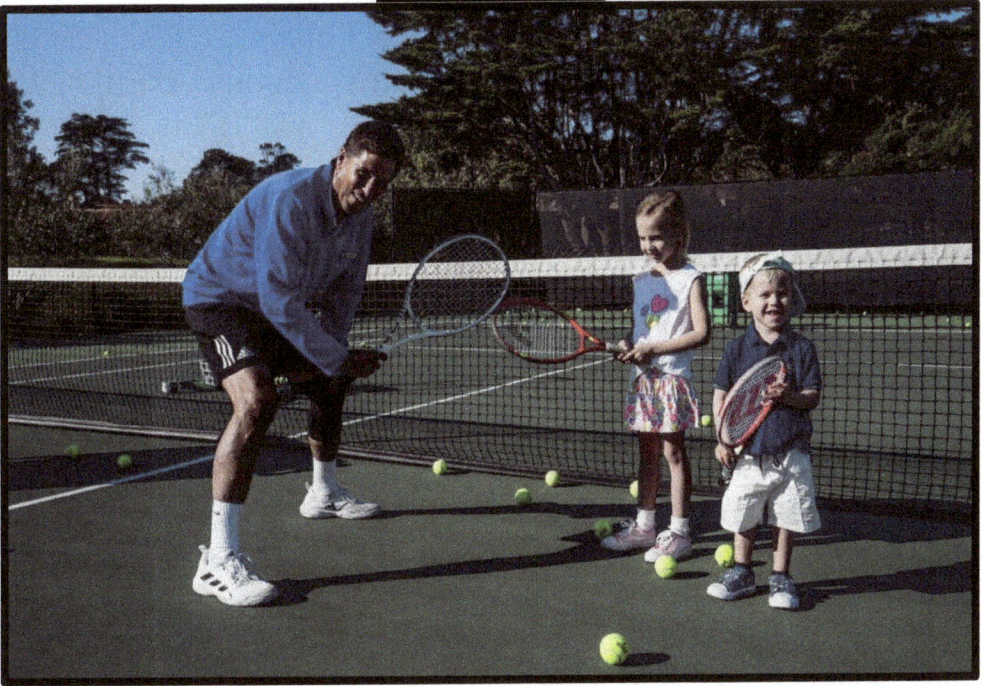

A Clear, Simple, and Knowledgeable Handbook for Parents Who Believe All Schooling Should Start After 24 Months

ded'i-ca'tion

Albert Einstein (1879 – 1955), an American (German-Born) physicist who never played any type of organized sport, said, "If you can't explain it simply, you don't understand it well enough yourself."

Since the first edition of "Lawn Tennis" by Walter Clopton Wingfield was published during February 1874, the first of its kind in the 150-year history of tennis literature, thousands upon thousands of books have been published in the English-speaking countries advertising moderately uncomplicated and elementary instructional guides, some even selling to the unaware beginner dramatic fatuous methods how the game should be played, taught, and enjoyed.

Every net and mid-court position, service and baseline movement, and stroke by stroke swing each writer wrote about was claimed to be exceptionally well researched and played by the writer himself to not only best guide beginners, but also prospective lawn tennis high school instructors and college coaches serving their students with the help they needed. Occasionally an author dared reinforce the notion that if properly taught the game of tennis was relatively simple-easy to learn.

Now, the co-authors of this compendium note two impassioned tennis-teaching young women who soared with their meaningful and popular instruction in the late 1920s.

Helen Irene Driver, a Ph.D. Consultant in Mental Hygiene and Group Therapy, was Head of Tennis Instruction in the University of Wisconsin's Physical Education Department. Year after year, free of her teaching responsibilities when the academic year ended, she devoted her summer vacation to week-long sessions instructing P. E. faculties on how to teach tennis at a variety of colleges and universities across America and Sweden. In 1936, this fabulous woman, already acclaimed by the U.S. Lawn Tennis Association, among a host of other national and foreign tennis organizations, including some in the USSR, wrote the popular guide, "Tennis for Teachers" (W.B. Saunders Company), which sold during years that followed more than 25,000 copies in 61 pre-World War II countries. The dozen or so editions republished between 1936 and her enlarged edition in 1970 was dedicated, and rightly so, "To my MOTHER whose courage and patience have been a constant source of inspiration."

The other spirited tenniser incapable of being fatigued hovering in the upper airs aloft the nation's rapidly increasing thousands of public park tennis courts was the pleasingly nice, gently humorous and agreeable, softly humble and modestly well-mannered, honestly accurate, and minutely honest and punctiliously, conscientiously scrupulous Mary K. Browne.

As the fountainhead of our continuing inspiration and resoluteness during the two plus years of often frustrating meandrous compilations and flexuous writings, Mary's astonishing achievements, not so much for her victories as a three-time U.S National Singles Champion; five times National Ladies' Doubles Champion; nine times National Mixed Doubles Champion; Wimbledon Ladies' Doubles Champion, 1926; and twice Captain of the International Wightman Cup team, but more for who she was on this earth, an ideal archetype of all that a woman is or can be. The fact that France's best, nonpareil Suzanne Lenglen, six-time Wimbledon winner, chose Mary Browne as one of her three closest and dearest friends was no surprise to the inner tennis world who knew both.

Quoting from Bill Tilden's book, "Aces, Places, and Faults", ". . . Mary has built up a fine reputation, well deserved, of being the cleverest and most advanced woman in professional tennis teaching."

For the co-authors, one in particular, a nobody, there was absolutely no other choice to whom to dedicate, "Tennis Begins at Two". A special gift from Mary awaits the reader at the conclusion of this book, one tiny aspect of her limitless generosity.

In 1928, Mary was pleased and proud to have her first tennis book published, "Top-Flite Tennis - - Practical Instruction Developed from Personal Experience and Taught Successfully by Miss Browne to Her Pupils". The publisher was the highly respected, prestigious American Sports Publishing Company of New York.

The first sentence of her Introduction reads, "In this book on tennis instruction I hope to make a simple explanation of the game, so that it will give to the average tennis enthusiast a clear understanding of the first principles of tennis. The most important task before me is to help you visualize the game of tennis, to see in your mind's eye what you are striving for".

Later, and throughout her lessons, she instructed, "It is in the simple directions and not the complicated reasons to which I wish most to direct your attention" (page10) . . . "The actual tennis stroke is very easy to acquire. Simplicity is the essence of its good form." (pages 11-12) "In all the years I have played the game, I realize now that I had overlooked the simplest rudiments of tennis, which are the foundation of Suzanne Lenglen's games. (page 118) "In conclusion, an examination of the point score of Suzanne's matches, particularly the important ones, shows that she usually relied on the simple process of keeping the ball in play until her opponent made an error."

In 1928, for Mary to have dedicated her first book publishing adventure to the actual GAME of tennis (a game at that time a fraction more than 151 years old!) which she so firmly believed, "Neither time nor custom will stale its infinite variety", was all the co-authors of this first volume needed to know. Both of us, from our humble, respectful, sincere hearts and minds dedicate all our efforts in creating the compendium to her.

We are convinced the tennis historians of the future will pen the exquisite play of Mary K. Browne on both the American and International Courts of Tennis as World Championship quality, then, upon that, recognize her foremost love of being a professional tennis teacher of tennis teachers. Her passing at the age of 80 in 1971 was marked by only a handful of sports editors who felt Mary was one of the five greatest women tennisers of the twentieth century.

The incipient forces striving for the conscious realization of her extraordinary uniqueness of tennis thoughts, the need for physical and mental health, and otherwise, including her motherly personality (married once, late, but no children) which was always evident in her work of TEACHING the young how to play the game, more than playing it herself, are certain to be reappraised and esteemed.

Her tournament and Cup victories were nice, and certainly wins to harbor and nurture with care, but it was her sensitive commanding the Wightman Cup Team girls with indefatigable verbal lessons, i.e., "Sportsmanship always proves one's character in its most courageous and gallant form".

Mary walked herself off the court and into the classroom to greet those who 85-year-old analyst Carl Gustav Jung (1875 – 1961), Swiss psychiatrist, psychotherapist and psychologist, termed the past, present, and future great minds in history. The "suprapersonal determinants", wise, intellectual young men and women who would possibly link her into each of their tennis lives and destines. Elderly coaches of sports champions understood what Dr. Jung meant - - and why it is we have so much respect for Mary's vision of tennis players and their lessons, thus selecting her for our dedication.

Included, nay, intrinsic, in our dedication to beautiful Mary K. Browne is a surprise gift from her to readers at the conclusion of the compendium collection: a complete, unabbreviated copy of "Top-Flite Tennis", hitherto unchanged and unpublished since its original 1928 publication and sale for $2.00 as her first edition. Several Copyright Records Specialists in the Records Research and Certification Section in the U.S. Copyright Office, 101 Independence Ave. SE, Washington, DC 20559-60001, ensured no additional registrations for recopyrighting were recorded or pending. Since 1929, "Top-Flite Tennis" has remained in the Public Domain because no publisher, no writer, no tennis authority deemed its spirit of lessons was worthy enough to renew.

This neglect included Mary's second volume entitled, "Streamlining Tennis", registered in 1940. If read, as highly recommended by rival writer Helen Irene Driver, the reader will find "Top–Flite Tennis", ". . . simple, concise, clear and well-illustrated with sketches and diagrams drawn by the versatile author herself." Written for tennis teachers and beginners, Helen concludes,"Mary's book as a whole is sound, as you'll read for yourself."

"Thank you, Mary, for our two copies", the co-authors smile in gratitude.

"Tennis, above all games, is slow of acquirement, and no amount of hard work later on can counterbalance lack of early childhood familiarity and practice."

--Mary K. Browne, "Top-Flite Tennis", 1928

Palma non sine pulvere, "Dare to try"

--anonymous

Occupation for Childhood

"The mournful wail of the little one going to mother half a hundred times a day with the restless question, 'What shall I do?' merely voices the cry of all childhood for occupation and presents to parents a problem which needs to be solved anew with each new day. That part of the thought and care of the mother which is given to directing the recreations of childhood as to render them fresh and attractive, and at the same time educational in their tendency, is wisely used. Children need variety of play, as well as of study or work, and are happiest when they can find it in the line of construction or investigation. The building of a snow fort, and the observation of a spider's web in a sunny window corner, will, each in its own way, interest, amuse, and educate a family of children. But no single suggestion from the mother will fill up the whole morning, or all the afternoon. Fertility of invention, constant interest, and long-enduring patience are essential qualities for the mother who aims to see that her little ones are kept happily and profitably employed."

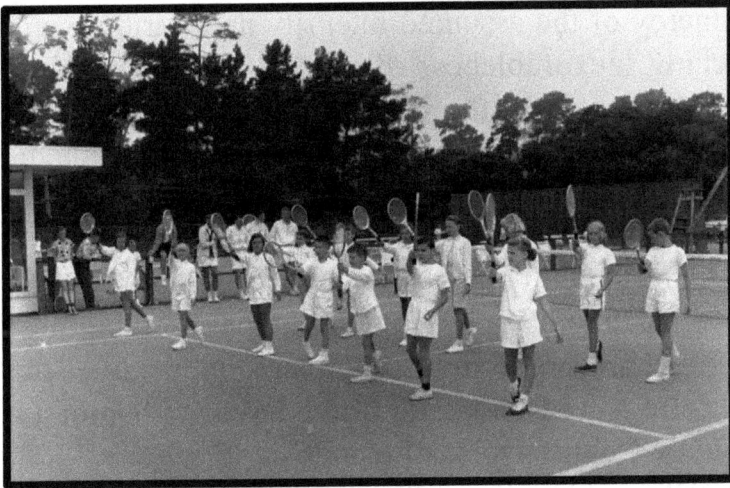

--Janet Clark, The Outing, Vol. III, October 1883 - March 1884. Home Brightening: vi, "Occupation for Children", p. 383.

Acknowledgements

A book of this range and dimension invites a collective endeavor of amiable advocates collectively cooperating with other sympathizing well-wishers for a common benefit. We were fortunate. Coming by good luck, bringing some not foreseen as certain, we were blessed with quality throughout.

Thus, is it with sincere, deeply felt gratitude we offer our appreciation to as many as three dozen California Pebble Beach and Spanish Bay Club members, friends, and neighbors for their thoughtful help in organizing the materials for this book, their constructive criticisms with clarifications of issues, and other apropos suggestions and time-consuming efforts.

Those we are indebted are referred to in the pages that follow. However, there are three we separate and single out, a library staff of seven; a 90-year-old tenniser, perhaps one of the best at his age range in America; and a happy, resolute, eight-year-old girl loving life and the game.

Writers of all literary genres sooner or later find themselves reluctantly before the mercy of the assumed integrity and attributive quality, ability, and unflinching inexorableness of a good reference librarian. Who will believe little Seaside, California, a suburb of Monterey, Carmel, Pebble Beach, and Pacific Grove, desks five of the best in the hemisphere; Dave, Alison, Amy, Carol, and Kelly, and two circulation staff, Nina and Kahor.

Then, there is Stewart Frazer, a 90-year-old spitting image Texian during the 1836 Battle of the Alamo, his eyes gently flashing the red blood of his pioneering forefathers. Immense talent commingling with his Lone Star nameless charm, faith in his own veracity, pride of truthfulness, and ineffaceable strength of body and frame have made him a notable legend in the Monterey County world of tennis.

And all followed by one of the swellest eight-year-old girls who ever drew breath, Juliet Elizabeth. Knowing where she was going since the day of her birth, no one can stop her smiling at virtually everyone around her and everything about her life. Upon completing each of Kie's tennis lessons, Juliet drops her racquet on the court and madly dashes to the court's corner to grasp the handle of the wide rolling fifteen-hundred-dollar tennis ball scooper. Now, the girl with an unforgettable smile is requesting one for either her 9th birthday or Christmas 2024.

Thus, it is with kindly and grateful thoughts of earnest, genuine praising appreciation the co-authors and photographer, David Day, recognize and acknowledge all who made this book happen.

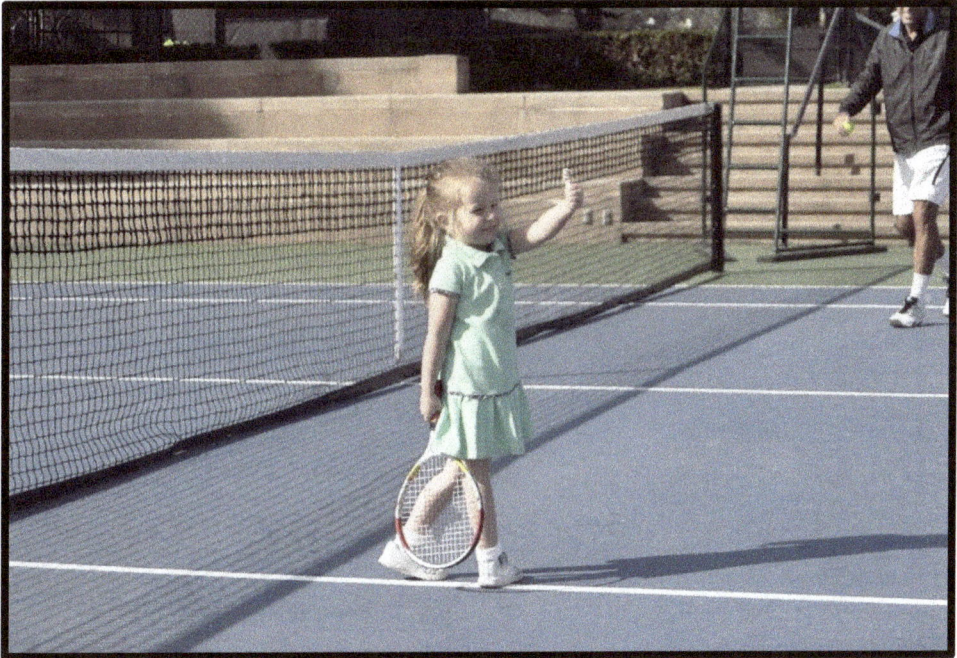

"If joy is absent while learning the fundamentals of anything; math, science, a new language, any subject academic or not, the effectiveness of the learning process fails and falls until the child or adult is operating hesitantly, grudgingly, fearfully at only a tiny fraction of his potential . . ."
    --*George B. Leonard, "Education and Ecstasy", 1968, P. 20.*

TABLE OF CONTENTS

xi

Prelude: The Romance of Tennis

by Don DeNevi

Finally, our effort, no more than an abbreviated but abundant and comprehensive cornucopia-compendium, is finally adjusted, cleaned, and arranged for semination with the parents of unusually eager, tiny, wee ones. Attempting to formulate a treatise of tennis inspiration points; long-forgotten quotes; tips and pointers; guidance and advice; personal questionnaires; all solicitous kind-hearted advice and achievement, on and off the court.

After more than three years of observing talented co-author Kie Foreman's on-court instruction with a then 4 ½ year-old, Juliet Elizabeth, of the rudiment first steps of tennis, we are certain that somewhere in the deeper strata of her awareness, as well as that of all young children, a voice has persisted almost from birth which in its own language continually whispers, "Juliet, no matter what you believe about yourself, you can try. And, maybe, just maybe, you'll find that not only are you good enough, but even better, that there is greatness in you for a richer and broader happiness".

Yes, our book is "ready", an adjective Juliet proudly and adamantly boasted recently when suggested being 7 years old. "No, I'm not! I'm 7 ½, going on 8, and ready!"

We begin with a passage from J. Parmly Paret's 1904, "Lawn Tennis - - Its Past, Present, and Future"

"There is NONE too much literature on the game of lawn tennis, as may be gathered by a glance at the meager (though complete) bibliography of the game that appears at the end of this work, and there is certainly need for more, since the game can be taught and learned by written instruction nearly as well as by personal direction. There are few capable instructors in America, too, which doubles the need for printed advice."

And, ever since, most "tennisers" have found J. Parmly Paret's words of truth commensurable with the cogent words of instructions, discussions of tennis facts, and game strategy principles in Mary K. Browne's warm and wonderful, "Top-Flite Tennis - - Practical Instructions Developed from Personal Experiences and Taught Successfully by Miss Browne to

Her Pupils", we have adopted their well-advised wisdom as ours. Especially that of unappreciated Mary Browne who, in addition to being a three time a U.S. National Champion, i.e., National Women's Singles Champion, National Women's Double Champion, twice Captain of the Wightman Cup, nine times U.S. National Mixed Doubles Champion; in 1926, Wimbledon ladies double champion. She designed for the A. G. Spalding & Brothers, established in 1876, the greatest woman's racket yet made by 1928, the hand-made Mary K. Browne Top-Flite Model. Introducing her book, she writes,

"In my book on Tennis instruction I hope to make a simple explanation of the game so that it will give to the average tennis enthusiast a clear understanding of the first principles of tennis. The most important task before me is to help you visualize the game of tennis. To see in your mind's eye what you are striving for, you need not know all the results of certain actions so long as you visualize and execute those actions accurately. Probably only one in every thousand persons who drives an automobile knows the intricacies of its machinery. The others know how to start, guide and stop it; for all practical purposes, they need no more. So, in the tennis stroke, if you know how to start, guide and stop your stroke you need not necessarily know all the surroundings and in a certain specific manner get the results for certain complicated reasons. It is the simple direction and not the complicated reasons to which I wish more to direct your attention. Then you will initiate action which will get the results."

Pivoting to the lament, "There is NONE too much literature on the game of lawn tennis... and there is certainly need for more since the game can be taught and learned by written instruction nearly as well as by personal instruction," from J. Parmly Paret in his "Lawn Tennis - - Its Past, Present, and Future," 1904, a review of the tennis literature then and today hints of the enormous popularity of the sport once the inventor of the game, Major Walter Wingfield of Her Majesty's Body Guard, introduced "tenez" in the British Isles in 1874.

If today, one was to type "Buy a tennis book" into Amazon's massive search-engine for its number of tennis titles, the return list would number 50,000 currently available! The two most authoritative sources regarding tennis book numerical counts published in Britain, the USA, and globally, are Books in Print and World Cat. World Cat is a globe catalog of library collections that enable users to search for articles, archival materials, books, journals, maps, music, videos, and other resources. For number of books published in America between 1883 and January of 1923, World Cat retrieved 6,389. For books published in our country instructing parents how to teach their kids above five how to play, according to World Cat, the number is 1,106. Under the age of five, the figure has never been available and presumed to be negligible.

Our book is largely the outcome of Kie's more than four decades of experiences coaching tennis at all ages above three, regardless of performance level. Our effort is neither a scientific treatise based upon antiquated strokes, positioning and strategic theories of great players no longer in the game, nor dissertations meant to argue one style of stroke over another, or to pose the question of whether tennis is played with the fingers, hand, wrist, full arm, or mind.

Conceived and created for parents and caretakers of the very young, our book initially prescribes a series of exercises to charm and allure children through the age of two to four onto the tennis court for excitement, dreams, and hope. The suggestions of the co-authors and their invited participants do not necessarily presuppose a playing knowledge of the game, its first steps or initial principles.

At present, as far as it is known, there has never been, nor is there today, a work of tennis instruction for parents of two-year-olds to address, adapt, and adhere to as the core of their teaching. The books of well-known players or critics of the game as far as is recognized, dare not embroil themselves in the controversy whether two-year olds are too young to fall in love with romance of a sport. The co-authors recognize and appreciate with humble diffidence theirs is a temporary expedient until something better comes along.

"Meet Kie, your new instructor."

by co-author Don DeNevi

"The secret of all good tennis coaching? Try approaching every child as a worthy, rising new star . . ."

--Kie Foreman, Director of Tennis, Beach & Tennis Club at the Lodge at Pebble Beach.

"Isn't my Juliet beautiful out there on the teaching court?", beamed Christy, Juliet's mom, as I sat beside her among the family, all of us mesmerized by how engaged her daughter was rallying with Kie. "Unadorned balanced proportions with grace, radiance, and elegance, all flowing from a three-year-old frame! Just like those kids, handsome and well-trained, in the tennis magazines." And, with that, we all erupted in spontaneous applause as Juliet smashed a two-handed backhand to the baseline causing her instructor to burst forth into hearty laughter as he quickly stepped back with a glance at the family. Scott, Juliet's dad, stood the longest, applauding the loudest. Juliet's grandmother, Nana, cheered wildly with waving arms. Simply put, I was stunned.

"Yes! Yes!," Nana hooted loudly, clapping, her hands vigorously and resoundingly, all expressions of encouragement. "Yes, like mommy says," Nana shouted, "eyes flashing and sparkling, heart glittering with love of the game; beautiful, for making us so happy with joy whether here or at home. We love you, Juliet!"

So immersed was I with admiration and my own quiet love for Juliet, whom I often refer to as a tattletale when she informs Nana and Mommy that I've teased her, I fought back a tear of total gratification and satisfaction.

But it wasn't just Juliet who causes my mesmerism. It was Kie who has a number one rating with the U.S. Professional Tennis Association, and is a certified member of the USPTA (P-1), a Nike National Advisory Staff Member; and Babolat Staff Member.

In 2002, I co-authored "Tennis Past 50 - - For fitness and performance through the years" with Tony and Mike Trabert, including Ron Witchey, for Book 6 of the Ageless Athlete Series published by Human Kinetics. Billie Jean King, Chris Evert, and Fred Stolle endorsed it. Although written

21 years ago and published the following year, there is little in it Kie and I would dispute today. "Tennis is indeed a true lifetime sport - - just ask any player over 50! To play tennis over the decades one will have to adapt to frequent changes. Obviously, as the body ages, strokes will require adjustments, in addition to being aware of new racket technologies. Kie had recently replaced Mike Trabert, Tony's son, as Director of Tennis for the Pebble Beach Company, and was instantly accepted and acknowledged by all. Not only was he a nationally ranked player, but also humble, a bit shy, and always available for consultations and lessons. In short, he was, and is, kind, gentle, and patient, positive personality encompassing traits which everyone recognizes immediately. Kie has the same qualities today, and even more of a "heart" for tennis, his family at home, the club members so than most of us normals who truly value and appreciate all he does for tennis, but more important, who he really is.

As for this co-author and friend of his, how he taught, and to this day remains coaching Juliet, proves so endearing that I insist Kie's lessons be shared in book form to parents all over the world in order to draw their own children onto the court with exciting home for fun rudimentary instruction before forwarding them a year or two later into the arms of the nearest teaching pro. Like his 11 tennis courts, 4 pickleball courts, the club grounds, his No.2 Pro, Bill Quario, his Pro Shop staff, the court grounds, always abundant with colorful flowers, nearby oaks and pine trees, the numerous deer living behind and in-between the courts, breezes off the Pacific, all seem to somehow belong and bow to him, personally. His club is his second home, the club members his family, not on the par of his real family, but almost, up-close, and very, very personal. It's not that he lives ALL his life on the court, but it may well be true he lives most of it within the perimeter and parameters of the club.

Okay, Kie, your turn – teach, as you always do, from that wonderful, spirited heart of yours! It was obvious that morning when you and Juliet walked off your Teaching Court, side by side. You winked at me and, when passing, murmured quietly, "Wondrous. No other words can describe her other than 'simply wondrous'. When I hit with her, and she's smiling, the sunlight around us seems to shine a bit brighter."

As for Juliet, she forgets all about tennis and immediately skips to the corner of the court where the manual 4-wheel green Metaltek Playmate ball-retriever awaits to be rolled out and around the court scooping up the dozens of scattered practice balls. There was absolutely no question in her mind that she knows where she is going and what to do with that ball-scooper.

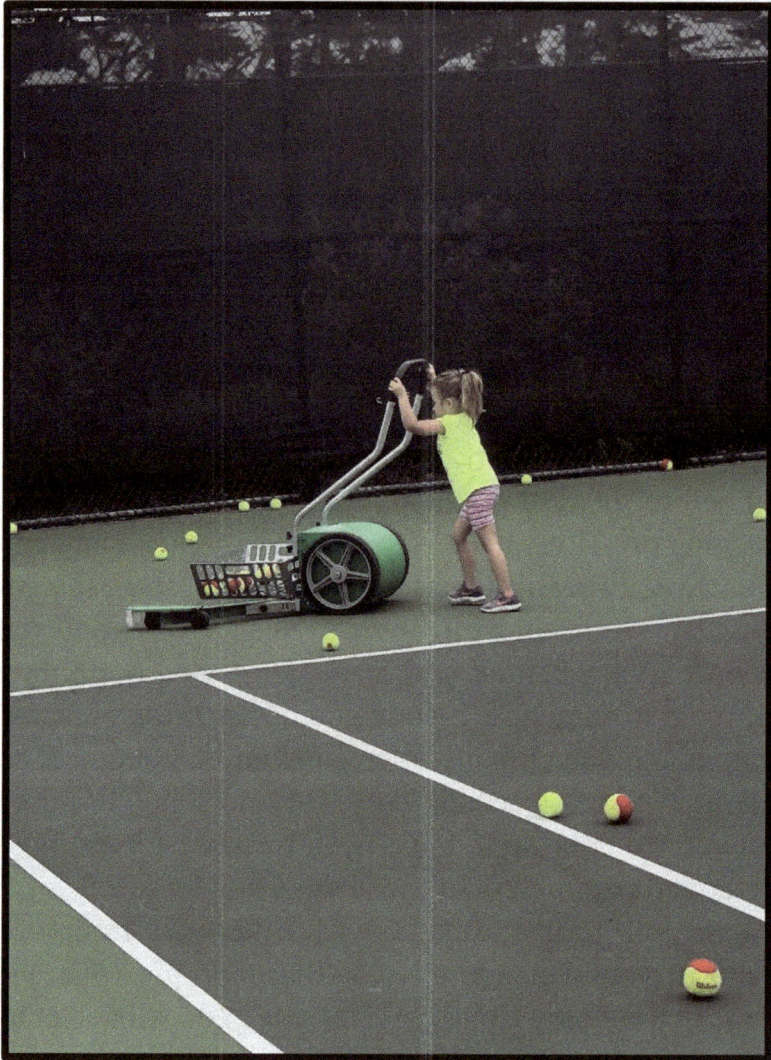

"All good and great people have had the will to win and the faith to sustain and guide them. Lying within us all are potential possibilities of greatness. We need not apologize for believing we can accomplish many things but rather, knowing the possibilities, we are apologetic for not accomplishing more . . ."

--Mary K. Browne

Three-time U.S. National Singles Champion; Five-time U.S. National Ladies' Doubles Champion; Nine-time U.S. National Mixed Doubles Champion . . . Wimbledon Ladies' Double Champion, 1926, Twice Captain of the International Wightman Cup Team. How is it possible NOT to fall in love with Mary?

Introduction by Gerard Issvoran

by Gerard Issvoran

'Repetitio est mater studiorum'

This phrase rang in my ears espoused by my father from a very early age. Indeed, repetition is the mother of learning and at age two it may be one of most crucial times in the development of a young child. Let's review some observations about what parents and children go through. At this point, Parents are beginning to see some landmarks of development take a foothold. Typically, life revolves around the mundane activities of feeding, eating, sleeping and reinforcing good behaviors as bad ones may or may not attempt to creep in. Let's face it, in terms of human development this is one of the most undisciplined periods of life in which almost anything can be challenged by an active and curious mind. That precocious two-year-old will have his or her behavior reinforced one way or another. The characteristics of patience, altruism, kindness, self-control, discipline, et cetera are hopefully being reinforced but are somewhere on the horizon.

The exciting and new world of a 2-year-old is slowly expanding but it's not that slow in the sense that it'll be as fast as those 2 legs and quick mind, will take that child at any spontaneous direction, whether scooting, skipping, running, jumping, or climbing up heretofore unprecedented heights such as the dining room table or kitchen counter. In my case, the roof of a neighbor!

As we observe the sharpening of the 5 senses that we have been given, those senses are even heightened in their tactile world of discovery. Colors, sounds, temperatures, as well as sensations of what is rough, smooth, soft or hard begin to take on greater meaning and focus.

If we explore further the breakdown of what a day is like, it is far more challenging for the parent to be able to keep a child in line with the repetitive schedule that most of humanity goes through and find structure during this precious time of discovery. The good news is that time will vary depending on each family's circumstance and it will be adjusted to each family's situation for their child to be able to explore and discover new experiences to appreciate and love.

Not to be underestimated in the world of our two-year-old is the hope and dreams of what his or her parents envision their child to be as an adult but even more so, the ability of that child in the moment of listening to stories and fairy tales of common individuals called to perform extraordinary feats beyond what they thought they were capable of performing. Therein is the fertile ground to take those visions and find a way of expressing them. By doing so, they will blend fantasy with reality as they see their young bodies with each day becoming a little more capable in a very large world around them. Those challenges that they hear about in stories to inspire acts of valor and courage are theirs for the taking if so inspired. But I think more important than the characters who are admired are the rules of engagement in those fairy tales that call out for honesty, loyalty, bravery, courage and a deeper wisdom in light of a perhaps at times a deeper sense of right and wrong, of not always falling for the easy temptation but striving for a greater and deeper goal. In sport, those same acts are practiced and carried out on a daily basis in the quest of attempting to become simply better.

Delving deeper into the life of this child it is worth it to break it down a little further. As a physician, all aspects of one's life are assessed and an area that must first be considered is what we do three times a day in terms of breakfast, lunch, and dinner. Having spent many years counseling patients on nutrition I will simply talk about the role of the three major macronutrients. In terms of fuel, carbohydrates, which essentially get converted to sugar and stimulate the pancreas to respond will give us about 2 hours' worth of energy. Sugary snacks will see our children undergo huge temporary changes and potentially explosive energy followed by the "crash", when their glucose levels subsequently fall. If a habit, their energy will go up and down all day long like a yo-yo and exhaust their bodies as their bodies have to repetitively battle fluctuating glucose countered by insulin. Protein as an energy source is more efficient and gives us fuel for about 4 hours and if high enough will also stimulate the pancreas to put out insulin to keep glucose levels from reaching too high. The uncontrolled level of glucose from these sources is essentially inflammatory to our internal organs, which is why it has to be regulated so well. If not, we may see the potentially ravaging effects of diabetes, over time. Lastly, fat which is a term that has a bad connotation, is actually the most efficient form of energy for the body. It can give us around 8-12 hours' worth of energy and does not stimulate the pancreas to put out insulin whatsoever. In terms of energy, sugars and proteins will give approximately 3.5 – 4 kcal/gm of energy whereas fat gives us a whopping 9 kcal/gm.

I mention all of this because if parents have developed certain feeding habits with their two-year-old, a food journal may offer insight into their behavior if their diet is imbalanced. Sticking with this concept of repetition, a regular schedule for these eating habits will perhaps help the predictability of energy levels for their child in anticipation of daily activities.

So, what are these activities that are emerging that as parents we need to be so mindful of? The mind of the two-year-old is not prepared to distinguish yet between fantasy and reality as everything in their world is so new. But if the concept of "play" which occurs with quiet time of listening, observation and asking the eternal question of, "why" then we understand, as well, the importance of balancing the quiet time with that of physical activity. Simply put, our bodies were meant for motion and the stress of that motion is what builds strength, endurance, coordination, and enjoyment if positively reinforced.

During this period of growth for our two-year-old, we cannot underestimate the value of rest. Without rest, there is no proper growth, literally. So, while we strive for "regular" hours of breakfast, lunch and dinner, we also need to observe those regular hours of sleep and nap time. As parents, we know that no two siblings follow the exact same patterns of sleep, despite the same parents and genetic makeup. Nothing is better than a refreshed mind and good mood after a nap. Nothing is worse than a tired and cranky child who has been taken out of his or her routine and will let all in shouting distance know about it!

All of this is to say that as we understand these daily patterns which vary from family to family, we nevertheless send our child into a world of predictive patterns that create an anticipation of activities that set both the parent and child into a routine that can be fairly predictable and at the same time is but for a season in the world of your child's development. Repetition in every aspect of our life can be easily appreciated by the adult mind but is also beneficial for our two-year-old prodigy. I am not mentioning the issues of hygiene and toileting at this point other than a routine for accountability can make life a little easier, simply because this is after all about tennis and why it is a game for life that can keep both parents and children captivated literally for a lifetime.

These are just a few words describing what can happen at this special developmental stage of life and having the privilege as a physician and parent to witness the incredible growth of children at this point continues to be cherished one day at a time.

"There are many wonders in our tennis world, but none more heartwarming and endearing and wonderful than seeing a little boy or girl holding a tiny, white-painted balsawood tennis racket . . . or, after a brief rain shower, four elderly ladies, lifelong friends in their late 80s, amid chatter, family news, and laughter, lined up side by side in a row

squeegeeing the wet court . . . or, an aging gentleman, our Stewart Frazer, in his early 90s totally absorbed taking a Kie Foreman tennis lesson."

--Don DeNevi, author

"After teaching my pupils tennis strokes and finding them lacking in self-confidence and poise, I decided to include in my instruction a philosophy which I know from experience can be applied to the game of tennis as well as to one's life off the court.

I believe within every individual is a creative power which is contacted through thought. WE ARE WHAT WE THINK. This power can be drawn upon as definitely as we draw upon our physical, mental, and emotional powers. There is a definite process of thought which brings us into contact with this power within us."

--Mary K. Browne, page 100, "Streamline Tennis", 1940, American Sports Publishing Company.

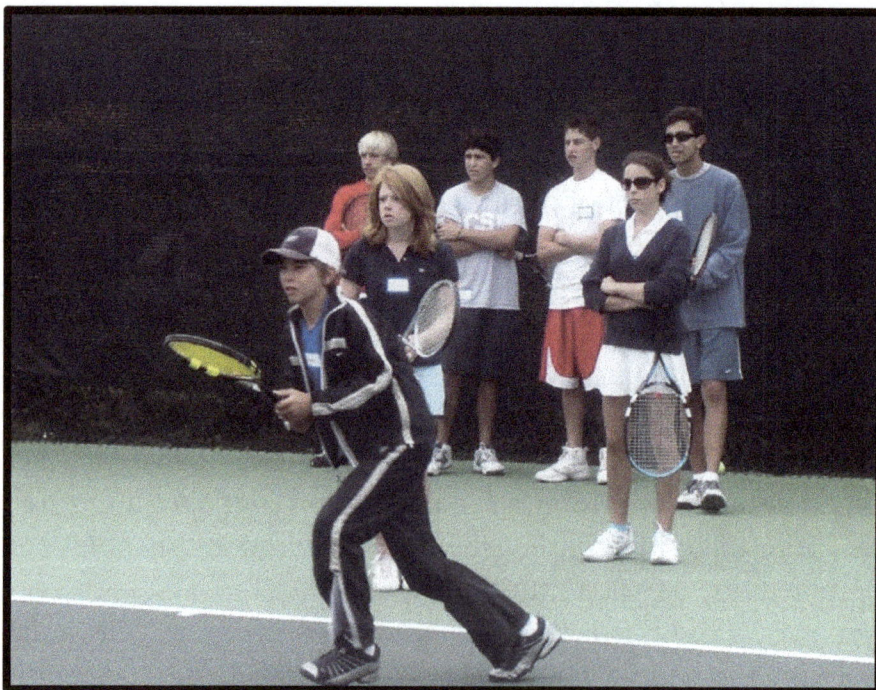

(Tennis Weekend 2006)

Chapter One

The legends of Pebble

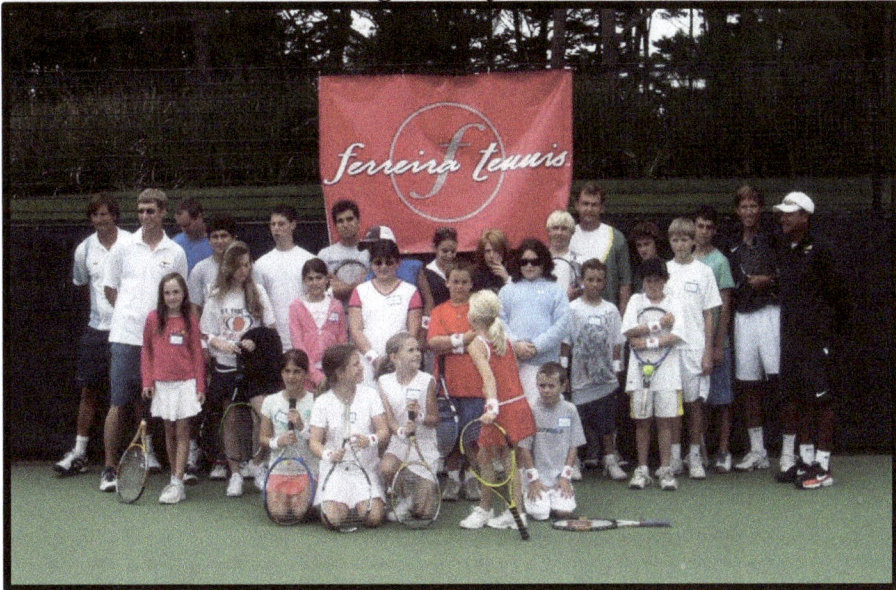

(Ferreira Tennis Kids Day at the Beach Club)

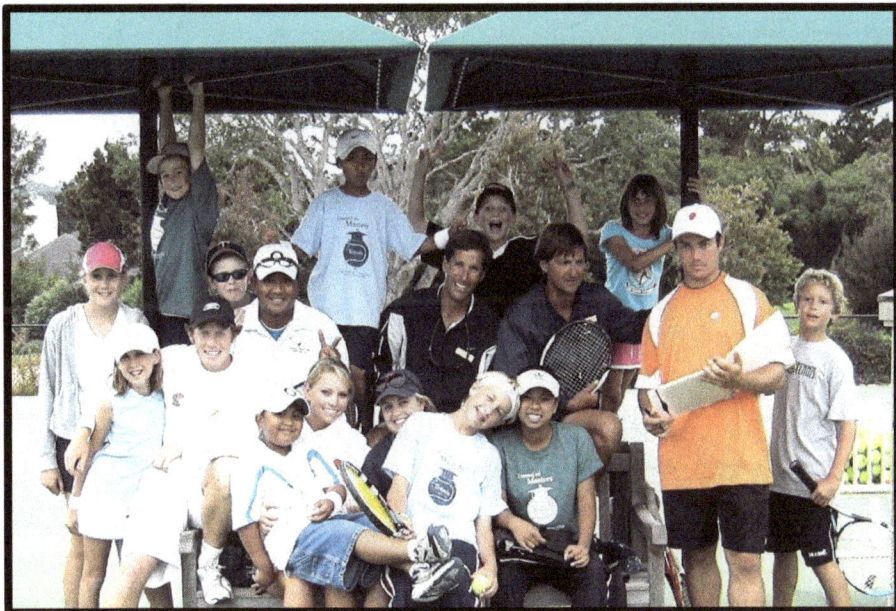

(Summer Camp 2005)

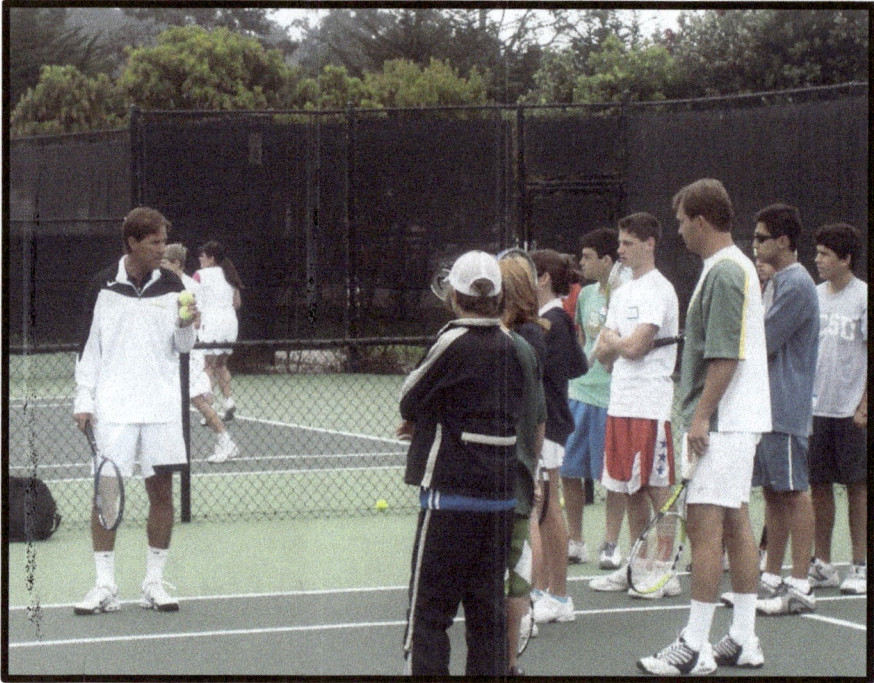

(Tennis Weekend at BC Tennis 2006)

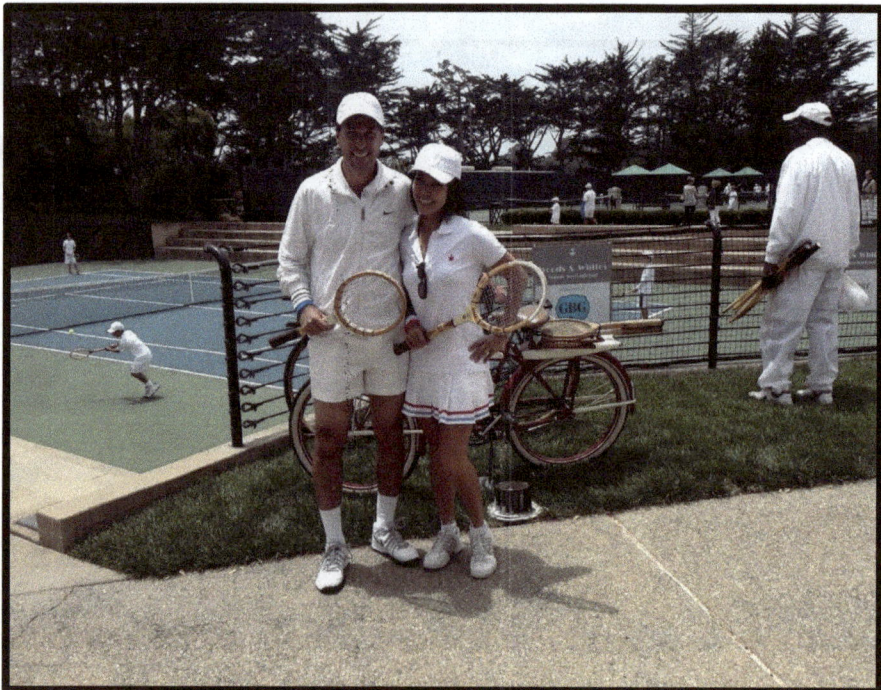

(Woods and Whites)

14

Mom dropping Kleenex onto the newborn's stomach until baby, on its back, starts reaching for them,

Dad taping a small hand-carved balsawood facsimile racquet to his two-year-old son's hand . . .

Mom placing her infant in a backpack, bicycling to the court, attaching the backpack to the court's fence while she plays and baby watches . . .

While pregnant in 1867, and absolutely certain her infant would be a boy, Anne Lloyd Jones began decorating the crib with photos of high buildings and old cathedrals, for her unborn son Frank Lloyd Wright would become the greatest architect in world history . . .

Parental madness?

The coauthors think not--so unabashedly convinced are we that pre-tennis learning activities can begin while the newborn is still on his back kicking and reaching, two of the first lessons needed for tennis! So it was that we reached out for several dozen PC members and friends to join us in a unique publishing adventure hitherto untried, as far as we knew, the creation of a highly illustrated book entitled, "Tennis Begins at Two", subtitled either "Instructing Parents How to Tenderly Teach Their Children How to Play the Great Game", or the hoped for, patiently awaited, universally asked question, "Mommy, daddy, will you learn me to play tennis?"

As mentioned, there is at present no book on the market, nor has there ever been a book published, a book on instructing parents how to teach two-year-old children how to play the game by anyone, well-known players, on-court judges, or aging weekend two-sets-only players. With great diffidence and lack of self-confidence, we offer this effort to serve as a fill-in for the gap in tennis literature until something better comes along. In a way, it is also intended as a means to appreciate some of the best who ever played the game.

This allotted portion of our book has been reserved for the specific purpose of hearing from members of our Pebble Beach Tennis and Swim Club. Most of these interesting, nay, inspiring accounts were written by life-long veterans of the game, male and female, because the premise of our book inspired them to do so. For us, the co-authors, to read and enjoy without editing or making a single correction has been the peak of experiences, other than observe Kie with the kids on the court. In addition, we were pleased the writers were cognizant, due to our need for cogency, of the book's limited spaciousness. Note, not one of the contributors is a professional writer, although his or her story is compellingly narrated. Not one essay lacks clarity. Each, eager to assist, took the time to sit down and share his or her story or party. Knowing most of them personally, we can say the essays are sincerely commensurable with the personalities who wrote them.

A Proud Sampling of the Pebble Legends

It was with much frustration that from the many recognized as such who we wished to include, none were available, undoubtably due to modesty and diffidence.

Fortunately, not all got away. The group we've assembled here will appeal to the majority, especially the aspiring young, due to their obvious unadulterated, unalterable love of the sport. For the coauthors, it's been exciting to learn so many unknown interesting facets of the backgrounds of our friends and fellow club members, especially what brought them to the game we all enjoy so much.

Bill Quario

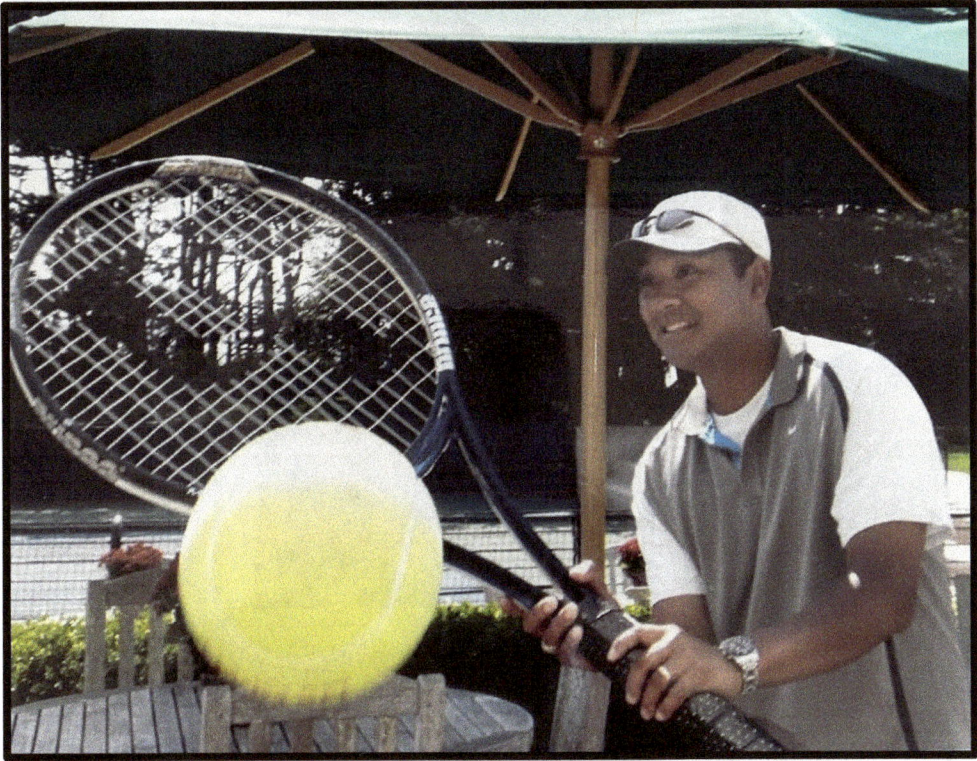

(Bill Quario, recently, with oversize racquet demonstrating the first lesson in tennis -- "Not only watch the ball hit the racquet but try to follow it AFTER you've hit it as you resume your normal position.")

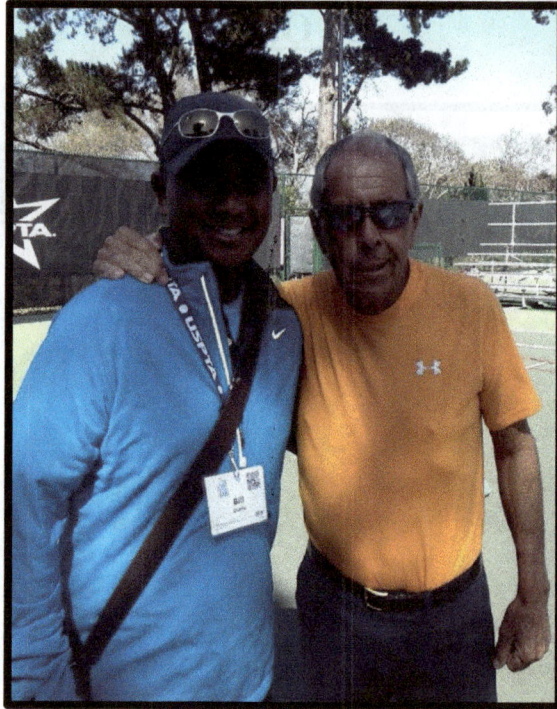

(One of the great coaches in the history of tennis)
-- Nick Bolettieri

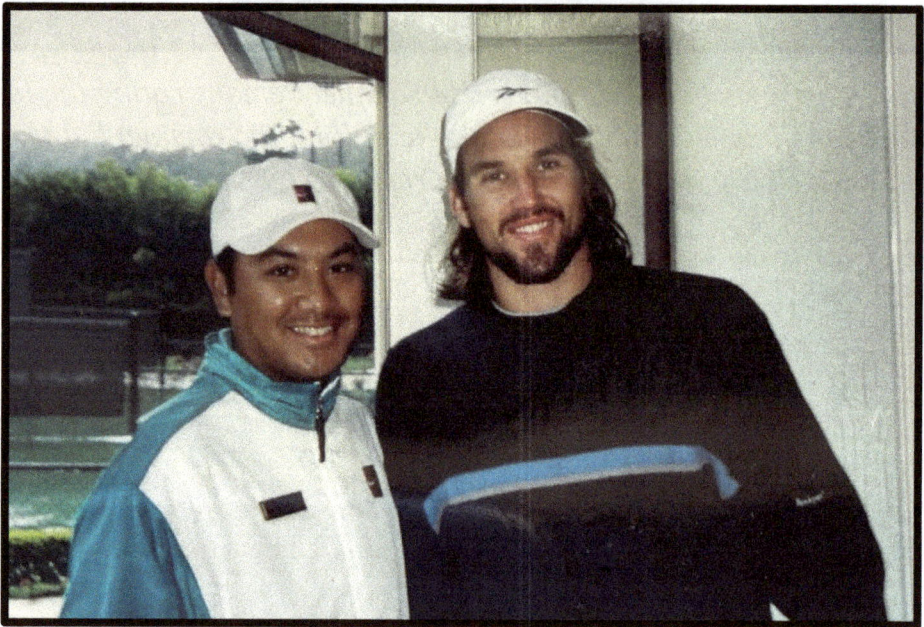

(Bill with Patrick Rafter)

(Bill in 1999, with Tony Trabert whose son Mike was the Director of Tennis of the Pebble Beach Tennis Club)

(A younger Bill, hired as a teaching professional in the late 1990s, in his office with good friend, Bjorn Borg)

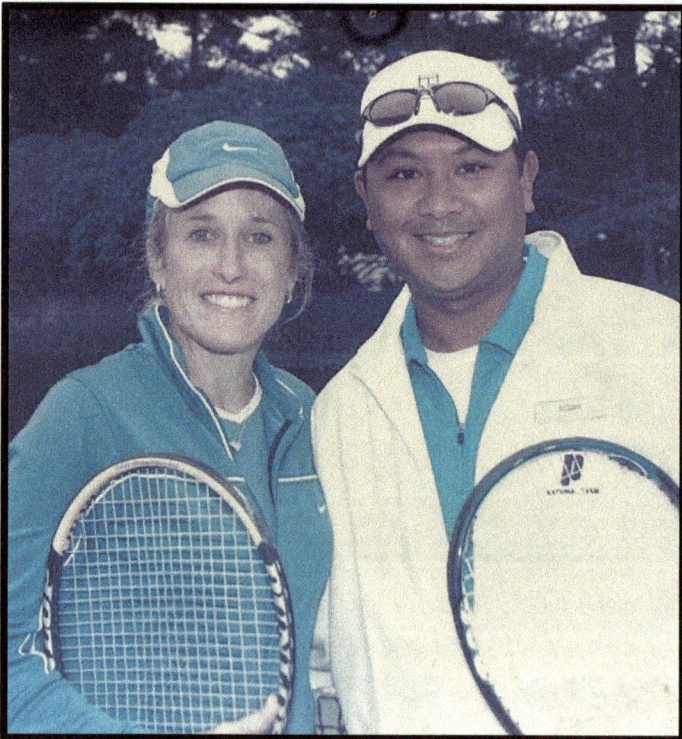

(Tracy Austin with Bill)

20

(Bill coaching Juliet)

21

USPTA Certified Elite Tennis Professional & USPTA Certified Pickleball Professional. He has been teaching/coaching tennis for the past 35 years and is currently the Head Tennis Professional at the Beach & Tennis Club in Pebble Beach, California. Bill was a ranked Northern California junior tennis earning an athletic scholarship to play for the University of San Francisco. His teaching/coaching career began while on campus at USF and at the Olympic Club of San Francisco. As a certified USPTA Tennis Professional, Bill was the Northern California "Rookie Pro of the Year" and a two-time "Associate Tennis Professional of the Year".

<u>My First Tennis Beginnings</u>

Having a father and older brother who would go out and play tennis on the weekends it was only natural that I would follow in their footsteps. After my dad was done playing his tennis match, he would then try to have me swing at a tennis ball that he would toss to me. But like many five-year-olds on a tennis court, I would just run around the court dragging the oversized adult wooden tennis racquet trying to just touch the tennis ball. However, being on the tennis court every weekend for at least three to four hours a day, it was only a matter of time before I began to actually hit a tennis ball with two hands over the net. By the time I was six years old, tennis became the one sport that I wanted to play and become good enough to someday not only beat my older brother, but also beat my dad. This is where my competitive side came from and led me to start playing junior tournaments both locally and nationally. Ultimately, I was able to earn an athletic scholarship to play for the University of San Francisco where I then began to also enjoy teaching tennis to adults and kids. After more than 45 years of playing/teaching tennis, I still enjoy the sport that has provided me with so many wonderful opportunities and memorable moments on a tennis court.

Coaches Corner-Tips to improve your game

by Bill Quario

Beach Club Tennis & Pickle Ball Weekly Newsletter, March 3, 2024

Are you playing with the right tennis racquet?

When the tennis club staff is asked to recommend a new racquet or demo the latest racquets, we will inform our members and guests about the three different types of tennis racquets which are: game improvement racquets, control racquets, or racquets which have a combination of both power and control.

For most club level players, we usually recommend racquets that have the combination of both power and control. These racquets usually weigh between 10 and 11 ounces and have a medium thickness to the frame. This usually allows the individual to still swing through their shots and not be afraid of missing to the back fence. Even kids making the transition from a junior racquet to an adult racquet, generally are better off in this type of a racquet, but with a much smaller grip size.

For the club player that is looking for a racquet that will add more power to their game, with less effort, we will usually recommend the game improvement racquets. These racquets are lighter in weight, usually weighing 10 ounces or less, are much stiffer or more powerful, and have a thicker frame.

This is an ideal racquet for someone who is just starting out, or for that player that has lost a little zip on their shots and would like to get that power back. Because of the lightness of the frame these racquets are more maneuverable as well. The strong, aggressive type player, who likes to take a full swing on their ground strokes and serves, are generally better off with the control type racquets. These thinner framed racquets which are heavier in weight, usually more than 12 ounces, allow the player more feel on their shots as well as more control.

Which frame is right for you? Come to the tennis pro shop and speak with either Kie or Bill and they can recommend a few racquets for you to try based on your playing style or needs. Once you find the right racquet your game will begin to improve every time you step out on the court.

Tennis Beginnings for Kids

It is always fun and exciting to teach a young child the sport I have a passion and love for. The first introduction to tennis for any child under five years old should be fun, exciting, and engaging where the child will want to come back over and over again. Through the use of colorful cones, circular targets that we call donuts, colorful lines that we call French fries, and multi-colored tennis balls, some big and small, I introduce three athletic skills that will help the child in any sport that they end up playing.

The three skills of running, throwing, and catching are all implemented in the child's first tennis lesson through a progression of fun games and activities like running through an obstacle course, throwing a ball to a target, or trying to catch a ball with a cone. Many of these activities not only teaches the child hand eye coordination, but also keeps the child engaged in wanting to continue to learn while having fun. As the child continues to come out to each lesson, we will introduce a tennis stroke that is learned by going through fun drills and games. Ultimately, the goal will be to teach the sport of a lifetime where the child will learn not only the game of tennis, but many life skills that they will use and need throughout their life.

Stewart Frazer

A true Texian

Thirty years ago, Christy and I found our way to Pebble Beach. We drove by the tennis pavilion, and I saw several gentlemen with gray hair on the court who I imagined to be Admiral Spruance (World War II Battle of Midway - task force commander of the fleet and former resident of Pebble Beach), Clint Eastwood, Dan Quayle, and John Gardner! I felt a yearning that someday I would be doing that.

My dream finally came true after I slowly worked my way up the Pebble Beach tennis society ladder and now I play with renowned Pebble Beach players such as Rob Galloway, Jody LaToutte, Stan Banta, Rick Manning, David Day, Ken Madsen, Mark Stillwell, Ron Faia, Don DeNevi, Jim Fuqua, Mark Fuqua . . . all Pebble Beach tennis champs, and captains of industry, each and every one.

Currently, back in Dallas, I have two regular games per week at Dallas Country Club's beautiful new grandiose indoor courts.

These current games were preceded by 35 years of being a "regular" at the mansions of Ed Cox (SMU founder of Cox School of Business) and Robert Dedman (owner of Club Corp., including Indian Wells, Mission Hills, Firestone, and about 600 other clubs worldwide). Ed and Bob are now in heavenly games. Club Corp has been sold.

The beautiful game of tennis opened all these doors for me. I never knew who would be playing in Ed's game or Bob's game. Literally speaking, it could have been just about any politician, prince, banker, or celebrity you could imagine. Part of the good fortune for me was that both Ed and Bob liked to win. In those days, I was quick as a mongoose, and my soft lobs and drop shots were well-suited in these social settings. Ed and Bob always picked me as their partner, because I don't look very good in the warmup, and this made our opponents feel comfortable. However, lobs and drop shots most often won the day! That suited Ed and Bob very well, because their other guests felt they were getting a better partner than me.

It was such a great pleasure for me for 35 plus years to receive a call from Shirley, Ed's secretary, and Brenda, Bob's secretary, to schedule those games.

After tennis, we always had extensive teatime, and the privacy understanding with Ed and Bob provided "lead room" non-disclosure of any teatime conversation . . . so much fun! This gave me great credibility, worldwide, when someone asked, "where do you play", I could honestly say I play three times a week at Ed's or Bob's mansion.

When Brenda retired from Club Corp, all the players had a great going away champagne lunch for her at the renowned Crescent Hotel. All the players were in a great mood and the lunch lasted for hours.

Any talk of Pebble beach tennis requires a lot of emphasis on the wonderful staff of the Tennis Pavilion. If you were filming a documentary about the subject, you would have to start with Kie Foreman. You would call "central casting" and ask them to send someone to play the role of tennis director at the Pebble Beach and Tennis Club. The response would be that they have no one that would be nearly as good as Kie Foreman in person. He is the perfect gentleman and sets a tone at the Tennis Club that is incomparable at any other tennis venue in the world. His persona makes even the most shy of us immediately comfortable. On top of all that, he is a great teacher. He makes you feel happy with your game. He gives you confidence and teaches without criticism, but with an abundance of enthusiasm. When he is teaching, you can hear him all around the Club giving his students extra encouragement to hit just one more good one. I have taken tennis lessons in some impressive venues, but no one can top Kie Foreman.

And Kie's wingman, Bill Quario, is perfect for that position, loved by everyone and always supporting Kie through the difficult times of Covid and the like. Bill is steadfast and steady as a rock. He gives inciteful suggestions and encouragement and he comes with the wisdom and intelligence of being a scholarship player at the University of San Francisco. Plus, his wife is frequently at events taking pictures which everyone wants to get. Bill taught me the magic of "bounce hit" and closing the racket just a little to keep the ball from going long. Bill and Kie, the perfect team.

You might like the red clay and the mountain view at the Grand Hotel Victoria Jungfrau in Switzerland, or the beautiful setting at the Monte Carlo, or the Mountains of Stadt, but nothing beats the grandeur of

Stillwater Cove, the 7th, 8th, and 18th holes at Pebble Beach, the stunning Scenic Drive, and the ride to Big Sur.

But none of these Pebble Beach stories would be possible without the kindness of Debbie, Sandy, Ruth, Melissa Thomas, Melissa Woolley, Jeanie, and the great staff at Pebble Beach. They make the place run beautifully.

Wait a minute.

This book is supposed to be about Toddler Tennis. So this is the story about my son-in-law (the father) and his baby boy, my grandson. Before the boy could even focus his eyes, his father would lie down and place my grandson on his chest with both of their front sides facing the ceiling. Then the father would raise the Kleenex towards the ceiling and let it softly flutter to land on the boy's chest. As time passed, the boy began to focus his eyes on the falling Kleenex. As more time passed, the boy would raise either one or both hands . . . and later, the boy would try to grasp the falling Kleenex with one of both hands. As the baby became more adept at making a "catch", a very soft, light ball replaced the Kleenex. Then it became very natural for the boy to chase the ball as fast as he could crawl . . . then walk . . . and catching and pitching became a very natural thing at a very young age. The most important thing is to make the baby feel safe, happy, comfortable, and successful catching and pitching. It's all very instinctual and very natural. All children will progress at a different rate, and only the father will know when to go to the next step. This child became a successful baseball catcher, football player, skier, water skier, snowboarder, and a great golfer. His family did not focus on tennis, so neither did he. This boy is now a fine man and has now become a part of his mother and father's very successful oil and gas business.

Another story I told about Toddlers and Tennis is this: I played in a mixed doubles league tennis for a few years. One of the players brought her baby to the court in a portable car seat. She would prop the seat up against the fence and let the child watch. Remarkably, the child's eyes would follow the ball as it went back and forth across the net. It was strange seeing the baby's head go back and forth following the ball. I don't recall the age of the child. From time to time, it would require some attention, but the players were okay with that.

(Stewart Frazer)

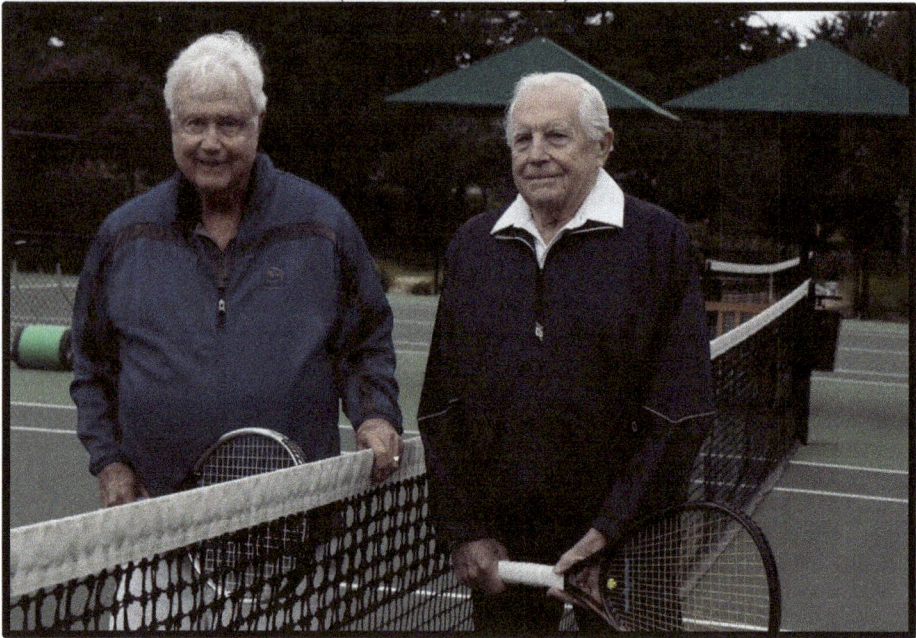

(Rob & Stewart)

(Melissa Woolley)

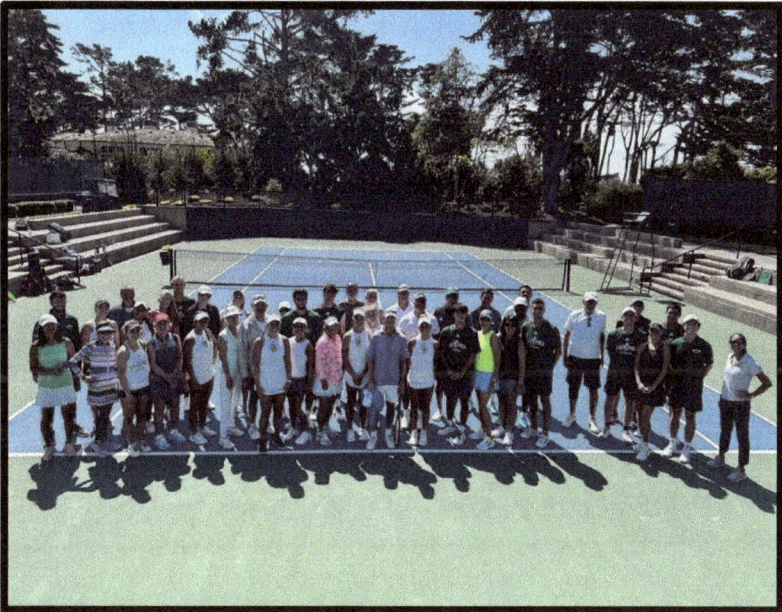

(Cal Poly Fundraiser Tennis Event)

Well, who is Stewart Frazer, anyway?

In 1832, after fighting in the War of 1812 against the British, Granville Harmon Frazer, with his wife and children in tow, made his way to the territory of Tejas. He built a log home and barn in the forest of East Texas. He was a surveyor, farmer, trapper, preacher, and he made whiskey. The local Indian tribe broke into the barn, drank the whiskey, burned down the barn, and the house. So, Harmon signed up with Sam Houston as a soldier to fight Mexico with the goal of creating the Republic of Texas. They won that war at the battle of San Jacinto, and by treaty became a State of the United States. Texas still has the right to split into five states pursuant to its treaty with the U.S. Harmon received a land grant from Sam Houston for 400 acres of land in the Piney woods of East Texas. He was the father of ten children, and I came along five generations later.

In 1933, I was born in the Humble Oil and Refinery company clinic in Baytown, TX. I graduated from the University of Texas and was immediately commissioned as an officer in the US Air Force and schooled my way through training, eventually becoming part of a combat-ready crew flying a B-47 Nuclear bomber in the Strategic Air Command. After four years of active duty, I joined the USAF reserves and attained the rank of captain while attending SMU Law School and flying out of Carswell AFB. I received a juris doctor degree from SMU and practiced law in Dallas for 56 years. I am still licensed to practice law in state and federal court in Texas, the US 5th Circuit Court of Appeals, and the United States Supreme Court. I started playing tennis without lessons while I was in law school. I needed the exercise.

I have five children, all married, and 37 descendants, including in-laws. I am aged 90. I have lived through many wars and times of success and failure.

Now Christy and I are spending some happy days in Dallas and at Pebble Beach. We are residents and citizens of Texas.

U.S. Open Story

My obituary will truthfully state: Stewart made the third round of the qualifying tournament of the U.S. Open in 2011. That year, the USTA set up qualifying tournaments in about 15 states and the winners went to a final round in Georgia, and the winner in Georgia went straight into the main draw of the U.S. Open in New York. To enter one of the qualifying tournaments, you had to pay a fee of $65 and be at least 16 years old. I entered the tournament at Beaverton, Oregon. In the first round, I received a bye. In the second round, I was scheduled to play the 16-year-old junior champion of Washington State, but his mother got sick and he wasn't old enough to drive, so he defaulted. Now, I'm in the third round. My opponent was aged 19, named Walker Kehrer, who was raised in Pacific Palisades and schooled in Brentwood. He took one look at me, and his gracious instincts took over. He kept me in the game for more than an hour. Of course, the crowd, including his girlfriend, cheered for me every time I won a point. SO MUCH FUN!!!! I also had some nuns among the spectators cheering for me.

STEWART FRAZER TENNIS TIPS

1. Love the game of tennis. It will change your life.
2. Love your parents, your coach, your opponents, and your partners. They will love you back.
3. Play lots of matches. Several times per week. It will keep you active and give you a feel for competition.
4. Learn and practice lobs and drop shots along with the regular power game.
5. Stay in good tennis condition. Always act like a good lady on and off the court.
6. Doubles and singles are both called tennis, but they are played differently. Learn both skills.
7. The first few shots of the match . . . just keep the ball in play and save the winners for later.
8. Constant movement is required. Never stand still on the court. Keep moving.
9. Try to anticipate what your opponent will do next.

10. Change your game constantly so your opponent will never be sure what you will do.
11. Hit the ball in front of you . . . don't let it get behind you.
12. After a long point, the next point will end quickly, so be ready.
13. Play hungry, never after a big meal.
14. Drink lots of water . . . be wary of dehydration.
15. I n doubles, play like you and your partner are tied together about seven feet apart.
16. Never criticize your partner on the court.
17. Play an aggressive game and let your opponent see that you will never give up.
18. Lob to win. Never hit a lob wide.
19. Never hit a drop shot into the net.
20. Be aware of the wind. It changes everything.
21. The first serve is the most important. Get it in.
22. Hit to the spot that will make your opponent uncomfortable. Don't hit it to her sweet spot.
23. Learn to keep score.
24. There will always be bad calls against you. It is part of the game. Don't argue about it.
25. Learn the rules of tennis and abide by them.
26. Keep a good sense of humor and laugh a lot during matches.
27. DOUBLES IS PLAYED AT THE NET.

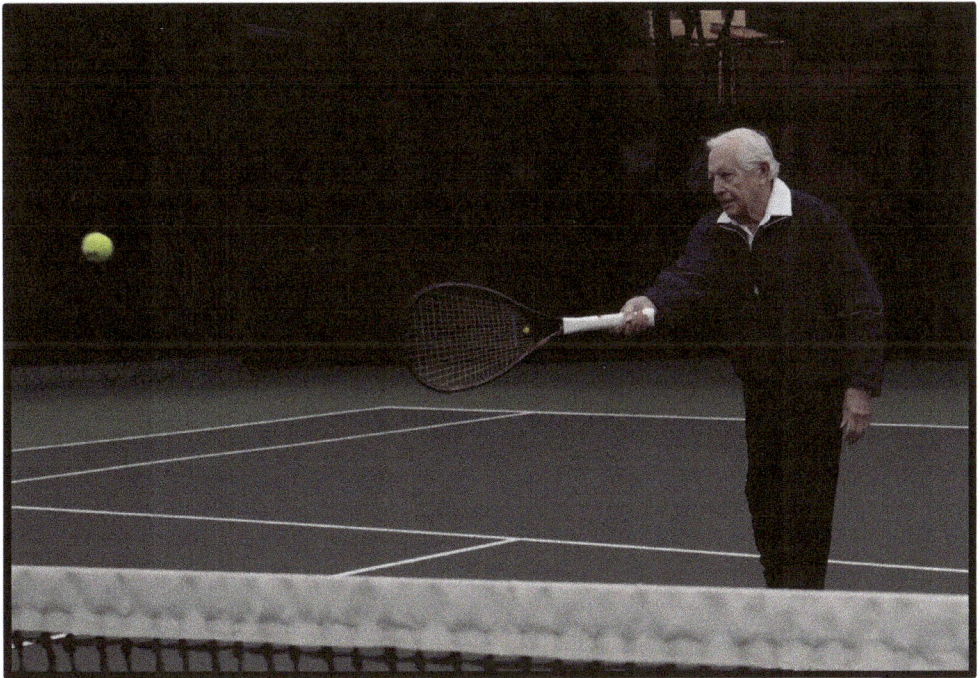

(Rob & Stewart)

J.L. Jackson

J.L. was born and raised in Luling Texas and other small towns in Texas. He moved with his family to Austin, Texas where he went to high school. He didn't play tennis in high school or college at the University of Texas. He achieved a degree in petroleum engineering and geology.

His father worked for Gulf Oil Company, and for a short amount of time, the family moved to Colombia and J.L. worked as roughneck roustabout in the oil fields of Venezuela. Roughnecks have a very high tolerance for pain!

After a few years he returned to Texas. He applied for a petroleum engineering job with an oil well service company after he offered to interview with the company president while driving his prospective employer from Austin to Houston. He got the job.

He gained valuable experience, and in 1971 became a consultant in a transaction whereby a coal company in Kentucky was acquired for $ 2 1/2 million cash plus a $ 7 1/2 million promissory note. The coal company was subsequently sold for $300 million. WOW!

While he was president of that company, he received a great amount of recognition for reclamation of land effected by coal mining. As a result, he was asked to serve on the Federal Reserve Board, Fourth District, in Cleveland Ohio. In that capacity he once again received recognition by hiring the first woman (Karen Horn) ever to serve as President of the Federal Reserve Board. A home run for J.L. Jackson. This all happened under the auspices of Paul Volker who was then chairman of the Fed.

Being a resident of Kentucky, he became interested in horse racing and acquired a beautiful filly named "Lucky Lucky Lucky". This horse was sired by Northern Dancer for the rather fancy fee of $1 million ... another big hit for J.L. Jackson. Northern dancer won the Kentucky Derby and the Belmont...two legs of the triple crown. BUT WAIT! This is a tennis story. J.L. played a little bit of novice tennis in Kentucky, starting to play at about age 50. He didn't have to diet or exercise. He played mainly on public courts. He belonged to the "Idle Hour Club" in Kentucky which probably involved very little exercise of any kind whatsoever. The Idle Hour Club, founded in 1912, is one of the most prestigious private clubs in Kentucky.

J.L. and his family moved to Dallas in 1983. By this time, he was President of Diamond Shamrock Oil Co. and other related companies. Naturally he was invited to play tennis at the Ed Cox mansion with Ed and his pals. You never knew what the "lineup" would be at Ed's house, but it was always a pleasant surprise.

Currently, J.L. Jackson is Club Champion of Men's 90s Tennis at the Dallas Country Club, and no member of that club has had the courage or audacity to challenge him to a match. J.L.'s strengths are: great serve, great service return, great ability to move quickly to the net and to retreat to smash lobs. And, most importantly, he never gives up. To win against J.L. you must play hard to the last point. Even though J.L. has had two knee replacements, he still covers a lot of court.

J.L. is currently taking lessons from Michael Jordan, Dallas Country Club Director of Racquets.

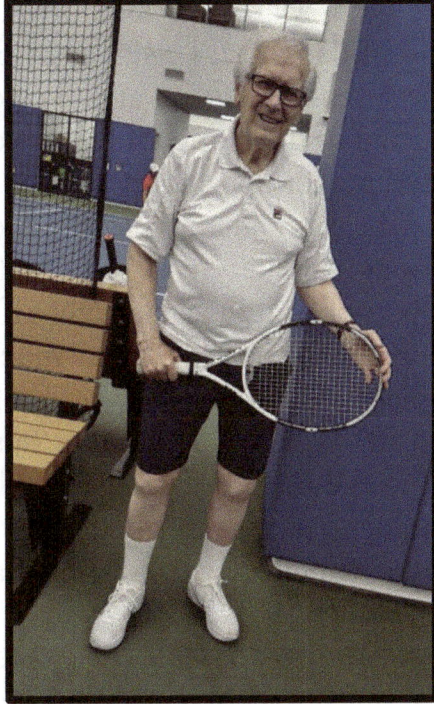

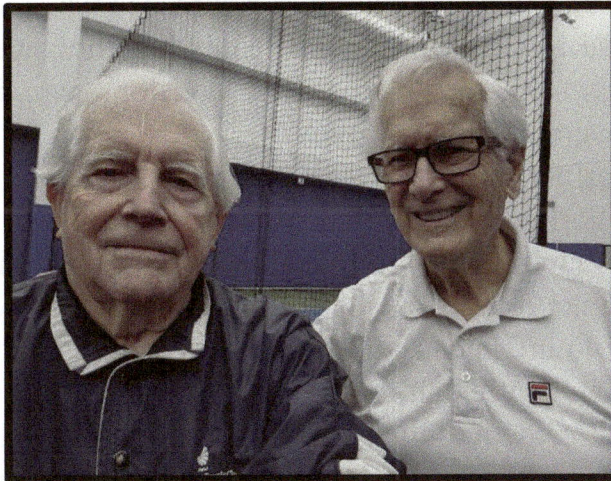

<u>Stewart Frazer and J.L. Jackson</u>

Lee Smith and Earl Ladd

For many years, my regular tennis partner was Dallas orthodontist Lee Smith. His daughter Anne Smith, who won several Grand Slam doubles championships playing with Martina Navratilova. Anne Smith was a contemporary of my oldest daughter, Linda, and both attended school in Dallas. Linda took a few tennis lessons at Lakewood Country Club in Dallas. Anne was dedicated to the game as a very young child; by age 12 she was an accomplished player and highly ranked in USTA tennis. My daughter, Linda, entered the tournament in a USTA event and was Anne's first round opponent. Anne was very confident and outspoken. She beat Linda 6-0, 6-0, and really rubbed it in. That event affected Linda's attitude towards the game of tennis, and she didn't play much after that; however, she and I won first place at Lakeway World of Tennis Labor Day parent/child tournament in 1974. Linda and her husband have had great business success in life in the oil and gas business. Anne Smith is now a tennis and sports psychologist and has written some books on the subject. Incidentally, my daughter Linda and I won the Lakeway WCT Mixed Doubles Championship, Easter 1979.

Lee and I had some success in doubles. He was left-handed and played with the longest racket I've ever seen. His lefty serve to the add court was almost impossible for any 3.5 player to return. He was a sweet Christian friend and we had lots of fun playing tennis together; we played on the same USTA team in the men's 70s division, winning the Texas championship several years in a row.

My regular partner in those events was Earl Ladd, and at one point in the early 1970s, Earl and I were ranked number two in Texas (as I recall) men's 3.5 level. Playing with Earl was like having a good dance partner. He always understood what I was trying to do at the net, and I never stepped in front of him, because I knew he was going to back me up. Earl is a great Christian gentleman, born and raised in Tennessee and rose to the level of Vice President of the First National Bank in Dallas when it was the biggest bank west of the Mississippi River. He was a better player than I, but he recognized the value of poaching, dropshots, and lobs, my specialty.

My golf story

Golf was my dad's game. He was president of the Goose Creek Country Club. He taught me to play golf; I played golf and basketball in high school. I never took to golf even though I played quite a bit as a kid.

We did not have a tennis court at my high school until my senior year. I made the traveling squad in basketball, but out of 10 players on the team, I was not good enough to be a starter. I had skipped the 6th grade so some of the players were two years older than I. We had about 1,000 kids in my high school, so that was pretty good. We got a tennis court when I was a senior, but the new coach, Leo Laborde would not allow me to try out. He said he didn't want to coach me for a year and then have me leave. He did not allow seniors to try out. Coach La Borde was a very good coach and went on to become head tennis coach at SMU for ten years where he won a Southwest Conference championship. He was also inducted into the Texas Tennis Hall of Fame, in Waco.

I often wonder what my tennis game would have been if he had coached me for a year at aged 16 when I was a senior in high school.

I never have headaches, but when I play golf, I get a slight headache on the back nine. Go figure.

A Stewart Frazer Story About Rob Gallaway

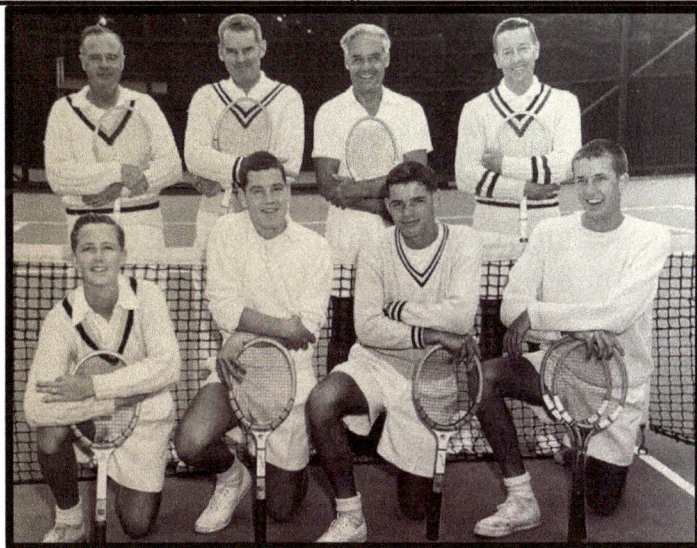

(Rob Gallaway- bottom left)

When I first started playing at Pebble, it was hard to get started, because my game is not pretty. I hit lots of drop shots and lobs. I had permanently lost one of the bicep tendons in my right arm, so I have to play using both hands on both sides. Rob Gallaway was the first Pebble person to recognize the value of my drop shots and lobs and he invited me into some pretty tough competition at Pebble. We played a lot with Stan Banta and "Big Joe". It was fierce, but great competition. Those guys were a little better than me, but my drop shop and lob gave them a different kind of trouble. When I played with Rob, we always had a fair chance to win.

Rob and his son Hunter own the Lafayette Tennis Club in Lafayette, California. Rob and Hunter have won several national father/son tournaments. Their daughter/granddaughter, Vivian Gallaway, is a nationally ranked 13-year-old player who is now playing in tournaments two years above her age. We will probably be hearing from her as her game grows up. She is seriously talented and well-coached by Hunter Galloway. Rob and his father won the Pebble Beach father/son tennis tournament when Rob was a teenager. Rob and his wife Pam are some of the best and closest friends Christy and I have ever had. Thanks, Rob.

Rob is a tennis traditionist. He was born on Carmel's Scenic Drive. As a teenager, he was a lifeguard at the Beach Club and served as assistant pro to the famous John Gardner. His father was a member of the Cypress Club and Pam and Rob spent many great times there with Rob's mother and father. Rob is also the current domino champion of the Capital Club in Monterey.

A John McEnroe story

In 1981, John McEnroe was playing in the World Championship Tennis final in Dallas Reunion Area. He was favored to win. I shared a box on the floor directly behind the player chair where McEnroe sat between games. My box partner was Bill Ward, a 6-foot 6-inch power forward on the SMU team. McEnroe was very unhappy with some line calls; he would come to his chair and smash a racquet and start shouting the f*** word. Bill's wife shouted at McEnroe, "Hey, Mac, is f*** the only word you know?". THAT made McEnroe even madder, and he got up and walked toward Bill's wife in our box. When he got close, Bill stood up and glared down at John. John turned around sheepishly and returned to his chair.

Teen Angel Borg Story

Sixteen-year-old Bjorn Borg and Ille Nastase were playing in the WCT Tournament in Moody Coliseum at SMU. My friend Tom Redmond was calling the baseline on the Nastase end. Borg hit one of his famous topspin shots. The ball looked like it was a mile long and my friend Tom called it Out! before it hit the surface. The ball landed about 3 inches in . . . Nastase's point. Nastase walked up to Tom and made a big gesture toward the crowd and yelled, "He is my best friend." Tom's face remained red for the rest of that game and the crowd roared with laughter. The referee then reversed Tom's call.

That is all.

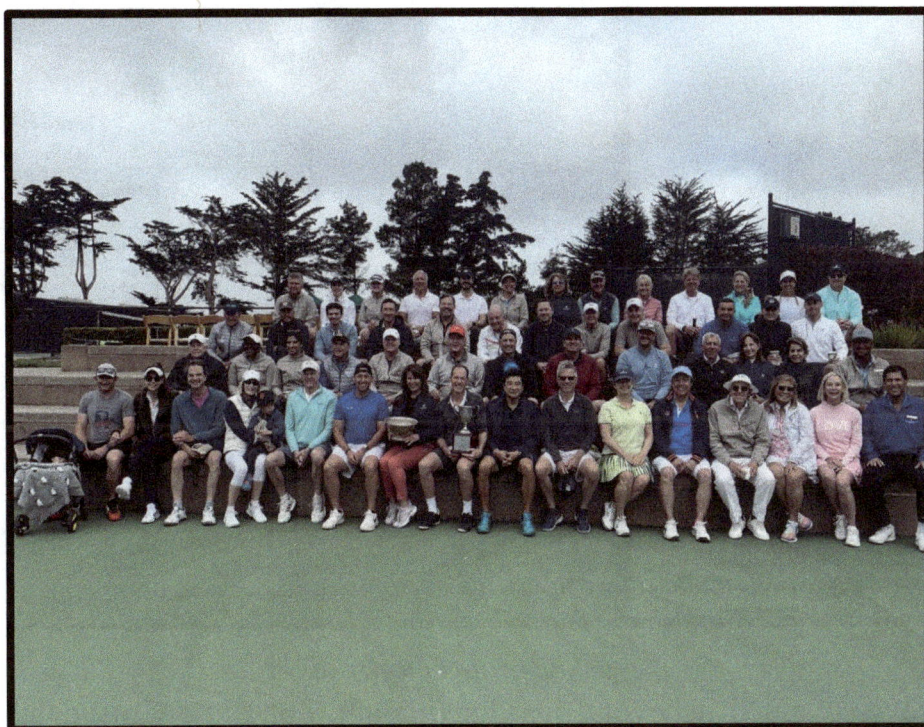

(The 59th Annual Don Bering Cup Participants)

Sharmila and Kern Singh

From Sharmila's POV

My dad grew up in London. He was a huge Borg, McEnroe, Connors fan - he used to watch Wimbledon and all the grand slams. Yet he never really had the opportunity to play himself. When I was little and we'd take family vacations, my parents would take us to tennis courts at hotels and we'd play around. I always got two bounces. Soon enough, my parents started signing me up for summer tennis camps at Kimberwoods in Fremont, CA, and thanks to fun coaches and memories, tennis became a lifelong sport for me.

(Sharmila Singh)

I never pursued it beyond just having fun, but I knew my daughters would (and should) definitely take it a step above - as each generation should! Kern, my husband, is lucky enough to be all-around athletic, so he played every single sport all throughout middle school and high school.

His parents also signed him up for tennis campus every summer in Fresno - so Kern baked in the valley heat and played tennis and still loves it to this day. From the moment our girls were born, we knew we wanted them to love the game as well.

Their first tennis experience was at the Beach Club's Junior Summer Tennis programs - and they've been hooked ever since. They both play middle school tennis. And every summer since they've been five, tennis camp has been a pillar in their summers. I am confident that my daughters will be able to play tennis the rest of their lives, and that their skills already surpass my own.

I always encourage my friends with young children to start summer tennis camps or lessons right away as tennis is a great confidence builder. Whereas some sports are solely centered around how the team plays, tennis is a game where you have to prove your own worth - and it gets addicting in a good way! Team sports are wonderful for many reasons. But we should also have the skill of being self-reliant and confident as an individual - that is one big boon tennis offers over other sports. Very few sports force us to challenge ourselves in a way in which we can't lean on a teammate. And although some might find that solitary, a lot can be learned from solitude.

But that is not to say tennis isn't social; if anything, it is more social than most sports. There are either two or four players and, more often than not, matches and recreational play result in close connections that you might never have made in a larger team sport. And as we get older, we don't need a huge social network just to set up a game - call up a few friends and you get to engage in an activity that makes you feel great the rest of the day.

So, for anyone who says they only love team sports - time to broaden horizons and take on a different kind of challenge! My wish for my daughters is to play high school tennis and to play for the rest of their lives. I hope they are like the 80+ crowd I see at the Beach Club - that would be a dream come true!

Gallaway Tennis Champions Span Four Generations 1912-2023

by Rob Gallaway, September, 2023

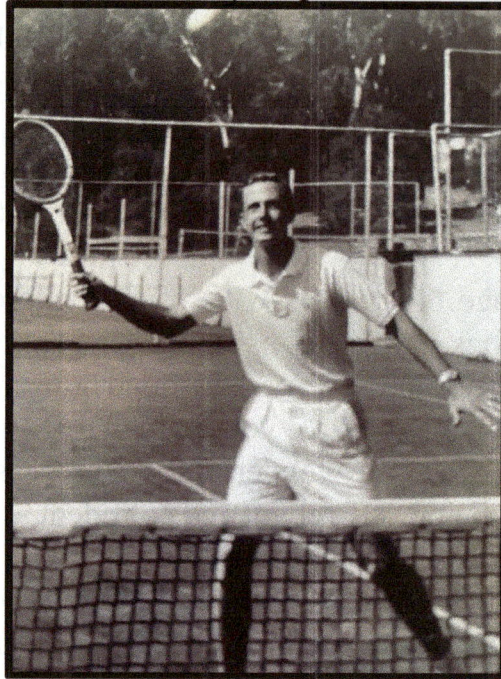

(Rob Gallaway hitting a high forehand volley)

It all started in Sacramento in 1950, when I discovered my father's old "Jack Kramer" tennis racquet and tennis balls in the garage. I proceeded to hit the old balls against the garage door, making little pock marks all over the door. I got in trouble with my parents. I asked them about tennis. We went to Carmel for the summers and at the age of eight, I met John Gardiner. He had a rubber pad with little feet painted on it to show how to step before I hit a tennis ball hanging from a string. I could do that.

I was blessed with wonderful parents who told me if I wanted to become good at something, that they would pay for lessons or whatever it took to help me. So I asked to take tennis lessons from John Gardiner, who had just been hired by Sam Morse to be the Director of Tennis at the Beach and Tennis Club in Pebble Beach. Mr. Gardiner was a very gregarious and inspirational tennis professional. Soon, my parents would just drop me off at the Beach and Tennis Club and at his summer camp at the Santa Catalina School in Monterey.

I learned three life lessons from my experience from teaching tennis from John Gardiner at the age of fourteen. These would be useful for the rest of my life:

1) I learned to show up for work on time.
2) I learned to be nice to people I didn't necessarily like.
3) I learned to use good teaching skills.

When John Gardiner started the Tennis Ranch in Carmel Valley, I taught tennis for him during the first year. While I was attending Stanford in 1961, Gardiner helped get me appointed to the Director of Tennis for the Devon Yacht Club on the tip of Long Island in New York. It was the best job I ever had. I was making close to $1,000 per month at the age of 19 in 1961. Being successful in teaching tennis gave me the confidence that I could be successful in whatever career path that I chose.

I almost made a big mistake when I as teaching tennis in New York. I taught a weekly private lesson to young girl, who had been severely injured and disabled from an automobile accident. Her motor skills were poor, so she couldn't do very well. I was about to approach her mother about discontinuing lessons. Fortunately, just before I was going to do that, her mother told me that her daughter looked forward all week for her lesson from me, and that it really helped her spirits and outlook on life. So, it shows that sometimes you can be doing a good job and not even know it. I cry every time I think about it.

My success in tennis was influenced by my father, Russel Gallaway. I later discovered that he was runner-up in the Eastern Boys Tournament at the West Side Club in Forest Hills in 1930. He was Sacramento City Champion in 1930. He was the Sutter Lawn Tennis Club Champion in 1931. He was captain of the UC Berkeley Tennis Team in 1932 and traveled to Japan to play Keio University. In 1956, my father and I played in a wonderful father and son tennis tournament at The Beach and Tennis Club. My father and I played against Will and Mike Gahagen, Ed and Tim Galwey, and Gerald and Gerald Stratford Jr.. There was a great photo taken of all of us on the Championship Court at the Beach and Tennis Club.

I played my high school tennis at the Thacher School in the Ojai Valley in California. I was captain of the tennis team, and I won the Tri-Valley League Championships in 1958 and 1959. In 1960, I played number 1 on the freshmen tennis team at UC Berkeley under Chet Murphy. Just before we played Stanford, I lost a challenge match, so I had to play number 2. This turned out well for me, because I was the only Cal player to win their match against Stanford. I won in three sets against a player named Chin, who was the number one player from the State of Washington. I had a sad time with tennis when I transferred to Stanford, because the coach wouldn't let me play ahead of his scholarship students, even though I was better. Tennis life is not always fair. I continued to play tennis at the Sutter Lawn Tennis Club and the Rio Del Oro Racquet Club in Sacramento, and the Beach and Tennis Club in Pebble Beach. I did win the Rio Del Oro Club Championships. I also played senior doubles in Palm Desert. I was fortunate to play tennis with Jack Bowker and Bill Demas in Sacramento and Graydon Nichols, Hugh Steward, and Jim Nelson in Palm Desert. My son Hunter and I also played in the U.S. National Senior Father and Son Tournaments, making the top eight in the two tournaments that we played.

My two most memorable tennis matches:

1) In 1957, I played tennis at the Thacher School in Ojai, California. We were playing San Marino High School for the small school CIF Championships in Southern California. The match was close. It came down to the fact that if I won my match, we would clinch the title. I was a sophomore playing a senior in the final match. The entire school, faculty, and kitchen help came drifting down the hill to watch my match. I won! We clinched the title!

2) In 1979, I got a call from Cheryl from the Tennis Courts that there were two "A" players staying at the Lodge who wanted a good tennis match. She asked if my son Hunter and I could play them at noon. I told her that we could play and that we would arrive at 11:45. They were warming up on Championship Court. They took one look at us and said they would like to play a set before they would play us. I told them that was okay, and that we would warm up on the court next to them, and just tell us when you are ready. They thought we looked like a terrible match.

44

My son, Hunter, was only 12, and I was 37. They were in their 20s. They kept looking at us, warming up, and they could see that we could play pretty well. They finally said that they were ready. They were actually "A" players. Hunter was so small that they could barely see him smack his two-handed backhand return of serve. We played very well and won 6-3, 6-2. It was a great Father and Son Match that I will never forget. We later played Senior National Father and Son Tournaments and made the top 8 in two of the Tournaments.

How did tennis save my son, Hunter's, life?

Sometime in his life, he decided that he wanted to be a great tennis player. In order to achieve that, he obviously had to develop discipline and focus. It turned him from an angry young teenager to a young man with discipline to accomplish his tennis goals.

It all started when I threw him tennis balls to hit from age four to six. He got his real start in tennis at the great Gardiner's Tennis Ranch in Carmel Valley, when he was eight years old. He fell in love with the tennis camp. Rick Manning was the tennis pro at John Gardiner's who taught tennis to Hunter. Hunter loved the competition of playing tennis matches and reporting his scores. Hunter played high school tennis, but became better in college. He played at UC San Diego, then played at San Diego State for one year, so that he could play Division I tennis. After graduation, my father and I sponsored him to go on the French Federation Tour in France. He did quite well and won some tournaments in France. He came back from Europe and applied for the Director of Tennis position at the Tennis Club in Tracy. He did a fabulous job as the Director of Tennis in Tracy. He saved quite a bit of money, and I told him that we should look for a Tennis Club to purchase together. We discovered that the Lafayette Tennis Club was for sale. I decided that purchasing it would be relatively safe because of the high value of the land in the East Bay, and because of Hunter's tennis teaching skills. We purchased the Club together in 1999. The Club was on three and a half acres, had 9 courts, six of which were lit, a large clubhouse, locker rooms, and a swimming pool. He went on to make a great success of the Lafayette Tennis Club. The USPTA awarded Hunter the "Best Director or Tennis in the United States" in 2020.

Hunter was able to improve his tennis from age 30 to 40. I was able to watch him win his first Gold Ball and National Title in the U.S. National 35 Indoors in Overland Park, Kansas. He went on to win many other Gold, Silver, and Bronze Balls in the U.S. 35s and 40s. However, his biggest accomplishment was to represent the United States on four different Senior Cup Teams. He played for the United States in Turkey, Australia, South Africa, and Spain. If he played in the National Senior Tournaments today, he would probably be in the top four in the United States.

His oldest daughter, Vivian, who is only 16, has won many titles and plays in the National Junior Tournament all over the United States. This involves a lot of travel and expense. She is probably playing well enough to be offered a Division I Scholarship. All of my other four grandchildren play tennis.

My involvement with tennis led to many different business opportunities in my real estate career. I became good friends with Bill Campbell who owned the tennis club, Rio Del Oro, that was right next to my real estate office in Sacramento. He ended up owning 10 different tennis clubs through his company, Spare Time, Inc. His wife, Margie, became president of the Northern California Tennis Association. Bill and I did three very successful real estate joint ventures together in Sacramento and Woodland.

Lifelong friendships made through tennis:

I guess that I would have to start with my brother, Alan, as he played competitive tennis all of his life. While I was in college, and he was living in Florence, Italy, my parents funded a trip for six weeks for us to travel all over Europe. We played tennis almost every day during our travels. We would drive into new towns and find the tennis club and pay the fees to play tennis. Towards the end of our trip, I finally got better and beat him in Vienna. I was happy to discover that my brother Alan's daughter, Rita, had rediscovered tennis, and plays for the Olympic Club in San Francisco, when they play the Bering Cup at the Beach and Tennis Club.

I have had a lot of friendships from tennis in Sacramento with Bill Campbell, Bill Demas, Jack Bowker, and Ron Rott. At the Beach and Tennis Club, I developed friendships with Suzi Crary, Don Butts, Ron

Lowell, Stan Banta, and many others. I still have great memories of playing tennis with Graydon Nichols, Hugh Stewart, and Jim Nelson in the Desert. I have recently met a wonderful player, Stewart Frazer, from Dallas Texas, who plays at the Beach Club. Since I switches to doubles, I always met three new friends.

The Gallaway family has been blessed with four generations of competitive tennis players. I wish every family in the future to have the good fortune to discover the wonders of tennis.

I will close with a copy of a poem about tennis that I wrote when I was sixteen years old, entitled "POINT MATCH".

POINT MATCH

When my opponent only has to win
A single point to claim a victory,
It wouldn't really be an awful sin
For me to miss the next ball purposely.
Would I not end the heavy strain of play,
Escape the sun and rays of burning glare,
And end the burden of this fruitless day?
Or should I give this lasting match a care?
Is it that I should fight for every point,
And spurt with fiery speed for every ball?
Is there someone that I would disappoint,
If I didn't answer to the pleading call?
Oh yes, for I would really hurt myself,
And kill the very heart of Man himself.
By: Robert R. Gallaway

(Rob Gallaway and his niece Rita Williams)

David Day

David was raised in the San Joaquin Valley village of Visalia, California.

His first camera was a Kodak Brownie on which he honed his photographic skills taking pictures of frogs, squirrels, and his dachshund Heidi.

In junior high school, David discovered girls and did not take another picture until 20 years later when his son was born.

After about 10 years of doting dad pictures, his son went off to college and David began to look at the world around him and noticed the beauty of the Mother Nature and trail less travelled.

Today, David lives in the Del Monte Forest and tries to capture some of the wonder that surrounds him.

When not in nature, David tries to take a few shots of his tennis partner making their best shots. That can be very hard to do.

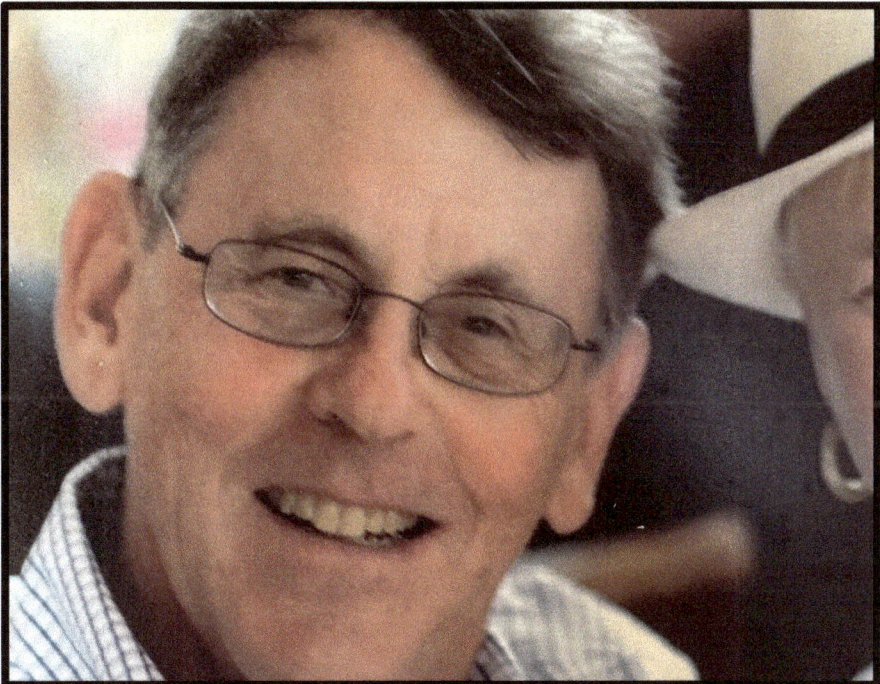

(David Day)

Betty and Walter Fink, Marin Tennis Club

My wife, Betty, and I were bemused, yes bemused - you could look it up - why a talented writer, columnist, published author of numerous books should approach us to describe in a short article what tennis has meant to us during our fifty-eight years, and counting, of our marriage. The bottom of the proverbial barrel was surely scraped when he selected us.

In desperation, "Short Article" may have been the key that turned Don DeNevi, the aforementioned author, to turn to us, as "Short Articles" could be an oblique reference to both of our vertically challenged appearances. However, what we lack in height, we are well-qualified in advanced age. As for tennis, we both learned how to hold correctly the racquet head in the crook of our arm.

My wife, over the years, has not been as obsessed with tennis as have I. She loved to swim, bike ride, and run. Early on, we were turned on to sport cars. We purchased the first XKE Jaguar registered in Marin County, and we participated in many tours and events, in both the Marin Jag Club and weekends, the Pebble Beach Tennis Club. Betty also owned an Austin Healy 3000, a Corvette Sting Ray, and we both had four Porches. Betty drove in Autocrosses Road Races and Hill Climbs while I sat in the passenger's seat with white knuckles clutching the grab bar. Our young son at that time thought that crashes, auto repairs, and insurance deductibles were the first lessons in Drivers Ed.

As we advanced in years, Betty devoted her outdoor activity solely to running, and loved the Carmel-Pebble coastal trails the most. She has accumulated a number of ribbons & trophies attesting to her ability and endurance in this sport. Gravitating to tennis as a sport dearest to my heart was born from various reasons. Unfortunately, heart is only one factor in promoting tennis ability. Long, strong arms and legs are a help as is natural athleticism. Being able to see over the net doesn't hurt either.

My family emigrated from London, England, and settled in San Francisco's Sunset District adjacent to Golden Gate Park which was a manmade paradise to a youngster. Our home was near the park's tennis courts. Because of my rather diminutive stature, I was seldom chosen to play football at Big Rec Playground. Baseball took too much time and track left me in the dust. But in the height of the Great Depression, I somewhat honed my athletic prowess walking in San Francisco's Financial District, dodging the bodies of failed and falling ex-tycoons.

As a hobby, tennis was a natural. The court use was free. Tennis racquets (wood) and tennis shoes (canvas) were relatively inexpensive. I remember my first pro racquet was purchased from John Murio for $3.00 after he won the S.F. City Singles Championship (the second or third in succession). It was a genuine Jack Cramer and the slight crack in its wooden throat did not prove a disadvantage to me. I started playing about the time of Alice Marble, a product of Golden Gate Park courts. She was the epitome of inherited athletic ability and strength. Her brother was a U.S. handball champion. Again, none of this rubbed off on me. I think in Marble's first or second year of play, she won the S.F. City Championship, followed by the Cal State Championship and onto Wimbledon. I enjoyed watching the skilled players at Golden Gate Park and looked forward to seeing Rod Laver compete at the S.F. Cow Palace. I would sneak into the stadium (part of the excitement was getting by the ticket collectors) and be thrilled by these two superb players: Power Finesse and Footwork. Maybe that is why my (and Betty's too) favorite art form is the ballet. We have been season ticket holders for the San Francisco Ballet for many years. The discipline required in ballet is, I think, akin to that required in world-class tennis.

It was a diminutive form of tennis that drew Betty and me together. Right after Pearl Harbor, I attempted to enlist in the Army Air Corp, but height was a barrier, so I joined the Navy. After boot camp, the San Diego Terminal Island Prison near L.A. was my first station. Al Capone spent some time there (with his cell door locked), Don DeNevi could or has written a book about him. On my 24-hour passes, I would go to the then-world-famous Ambassador Hotel where the patriotic management would provide the services deluxe accommodations for $2.00 per night, no tax. I think I was the only enlisted man to partake of their hospitality. And that is where I met Betty on a Saturday where she came to enjoy the sun and the hotel's beautiful Lido Plunge. I was by the pool at the ping pong table playing with a fellow sailor. Betty saw in me a pigeon and challenged me to a game. Modesty prevents my relating this outcome.

I was transferred to the Naval Reserve Amory in Chavez Ravine in Los Angeles which later was transformed into the Dodgers' ballpark. While there, Betty and I dated about four or five times and then were married on a 48-hour pass. Betty followed me to several radio and aircraft radio and gunnery schools in Memphis, Tennessee, and Hollywood., Florida until I was transferred to the Navy Air Corp and was shipped out. We were not reunited until almost the end of the war. The reunion which should have taken place in some idyllic romantic setting instead occurred in (with all due respect to Texans) at the Larley Naval Base at Corpus Christy, Texas. We were there until my discharge. To this day, I often think how Betty endured the discomfort, the oppressive, unbearable heat, the cockroaches and the hurricane she trembled through alone and isolated in the little jerry-built apartment we shared. The hurricane hit suddenly, and we flew all planes before I had a chance to call Betty two days later. Betty sat on the inside staircase by the front door which she couldn't open because of the strong wind. A dreadful frightening experience. This last episode plus the time I was away should have resulted in the well-known "Dear John" letter of that period. Instead, it is a testimonial of Betty's commitment and abiding love for me. A Don DeNevi would be better able to enunciate my love for her.

I digressed. There was no tennis during the war years. At war's end, we decided to make San Francisco our home. One son and about eight years later, I finally sold Betty on moving to Marin County - she being a big city girl from New York and Los Angeles; she viewed Marin as a wilderness, a what do we do if we need a doctor? The house we built was only the second on the block, but forty years later, we were in the first wave to join the then-unbuilt Marin Tennis club which has now been our home away from home for the past quarter century. As a matter of fact, various club Boards of Directors have had serious discussions over our interpretation of the word "home". They have questioned the legality of our assuming the club mortgage or, at the least, pay room and board.

Suffice to say, we love the club and, even more, its diverse members. The club is a magnet for attracting interesting, talented, yet modest tennis devotees. If one is willing to go beyond the "hello, how are you" and delve, one will discover fascinating personalities with vacation, avocations, hobbies, and esoteric interests. Your tennis partner or opponent may be a philosopher, a philanthropist, a practicing humanitarian or, of course, any one of the higher academic professionals. The only uniformity are the tennis clothes and the various levels of play.

The practical side of the foregoing is the economic advantage this has provided Betty and me. We need medical advice? In what specialty? On the odd game change sides, we can obtain a complete diagnosis - no charge. Same way to obtain legal advice - pro bono. The list of services is unlimited from animal care to Zoology, our club has it all. You may have to give a game point away as payment, but that is a minor concession.

Tennis, and our tennis club has provided Betty and me with a cherished group of extended family members that we hold near and dear.

As anyone can discern, there is much more to tennis than a power serve.

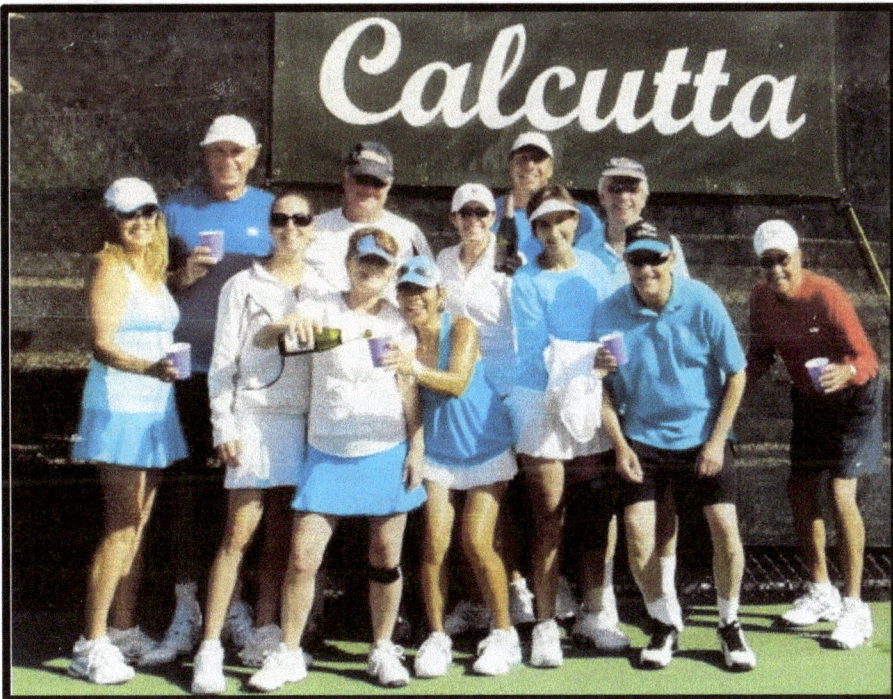

Kurt Schlesinger, M.D., A Holocaust Survivor

Throughout his career as a physician and psychoanalyst, Dr. Kurt Schlesinger has been probing the deepest layers of the human psyche, assisting his clients achieve maximum insights and new understandings of their neurotic illnesses.

Living until the age of 93, he maintained a full psychiatric practice in San Francisco, while continuing to write professional papers, present lectures, and attend symposia and conferences. In addition, he found the time to play tennis at the San Francisco, California Tennis Club and the Pebble Beach Clubs, two of the oldest tennis clubs on the Pacific West Coast, twice a week he played Marin; the Pebble Beach Club on weekends.

Every now and then, while on either court, he was found of telling his playing friends about the majestic movements of both the evolving human spirit (the goal of his profession) and tennis (the game he loved so much). Those who loved him saw clearly that Kurt was a perfect balance between an acute perception of reality and parapsychological experience.

Born in Czestochowa, Poland in 1918, Schlesinger moved to Germany as the war ended in November of that year and spent the first eleven years of his life there. He had three older and one younger brother.

Kurt graduated from Marshall High School in Chicago in 1937 and went to the University of Illinois at Champaign-Urbana, received a B.A. degree and worked on a master's degree in Drama when World War II arrived. He served in the U.S. Maritime Service in the Atlantic and Mediterranean theatre with the rank of Lt. j.g., receiving a commendation from President Roosevelt.

When the war ended, Kurt decided to study medicine and Psychiatry and went to the University of Illinois College of Medicine in Chicago. He interned at Kaiser-Permanente Hospital in Oakland, California and then was a resident in psychiatry at Cincinnati General Hospital for two years. Then Schlesinger spent a year in the army during the Korean War as a psychiatrist at Madigan Army Hospital in Tacoma, Seattle. He returned to psychiatric residency at Mount Zion Hospital in San Francisco, California, and later trained in psychoanalysis at the San Francisco Psychoanalysis Institute, soon a member at its faculty.

He was a clinical Professor Emeritus at the University of California, San Francisco, Department of Psychiatry.

Kurt has authored papers on acting out, Jewish humor, Freud and jokes, the creative process, ethics of family therapy, etc.

In response to the question of what tennis has meant to him during his life, Kurt wrote:

"In 1929, my family came to this country from Germany, thanks to my father's prescience about Germany's future. I was going on eleven. My father's younger sister, my Aunt Shirley, had proceeded us by some years and she took me under her wing. This included taking me to Humboldt Park tennis courts in Chicago.

In those days, these public courts had no nets. Players brought their own. Aunt Shirley had me help her fasten the net and gave me a tennis racquet and proceeded to instruct me on how to rally with her. This became a regular routine. We would do this one or twice a week.

I also played softball, baseball, and soccer when I got to high school, but tennis was my favorite activity and I played with people my own age throughout high school. I liked the one-on-one sociability of tennis over the "groupiness" of nine-person baseball or eleven-player soccer. The socializing was always much more important to me than the competition. I played with friends rather than seeking out opponents to beat. I played with girls as much as boys. From the time I first learned to read, I was an avid reader and the body movement provided by tennis seems in retrospect kind of antidotal to the sedentary reading activity.

I continued to play throughout college but had to forego tennis while overseas in World War II. When the war was over, and I went to Medical School, I resumed tennis. Of course, I married a tennis-playing wife. I have been playing for seventy plus years and play five to six times a week. I am practicing psychiatry and psychoanalysis and as in childhood, found tennis a necessary antidote to my sedentary and verbalizing profession. I am not planning to retire from either activity.

As I observe myself, tennis to me is a kind of dance, a coordination of rhythm and focused attention, which coordinates mind and body action. This chorographic emphasis is for me, a life-enhancing aspect in keeping body and mind coordinated. I consider how one experiences one's body a

55

basic mood determinant. It is true that there was a time when I played to win, and I have a mantel full of trophies from forty-five years ago. But it never took over and as I have observed these competitive champions over time, I see how they missed their loss of youthful superiority. I am constantly feeling that I am playing better. Better than yesterday, not as good as tomorrow.

I have replaced my angelic Aunt Shirley as my hitting partner, with "dancy" Cissy Harris, thirty years my junior and fast-paced Judi Walsh, forty-five years younger. They keep me going and I plan to play until I am 100 and then take it one year at a time."

Don's note: Although 5'2" in height, (it was really quite easy to lob him), he's considered a giant by all of us who play with him. Whether professional colleagues at Pebble, or Cal club members, everyone felt the same way: knowing him, and playing with, or against, him, brought a certain richness to our lives. We became wiser because of what he taught indirectly, more hopeful because of the legacy he inspired, and happier because of the inner joy and peace he radiated.

One of the more interesting, if not amusing, anecdotes Kurt repeatedly pondered and shared with tennis friends at the California Tennis Club in San Francisco, the state's first systematically founded by committee in 1884, dealt with an elderly Chinese gentleman sitting first row courtside observing four youthful tennisers executing delicate and power-driven shots of physical daring. Cognizant of the man as he chased a ball in a corner nearest the well-bred old scholar, Kurt noticed him wipe away a tear.

"Why the tear? Is whomever you're rooting for losing? They all look great to me, Mr. Hing!"

"Because I'm thinking, Dr. Schlesinger," he waved, smiling away a touch of melancholy, "if his parents and I could only teach my grandson out there to skillfully train his body and soul the same way the teaching pro here at the Cal Club taught him and others how to train his body feats of physical daring, what a wonderous society, and world we would have! What mankind could accomplish!"

Since that moment, Kurt claimed, he couldn't dismiss or erase, "Critical thinking coupling with tennis feats or other sport activities. Finding parallel cultivation in rigid inflexible bodies destined to be uncultivated. Strong thinking coupled with tough tennis, or other physical challenging sports, but always in moderation, and proportion, on the human scale. Kurt always taught his patients and friends, whether tennis playing or not,

"Always, regardless of age, wonder,

Always, question

Always, have the power to generalize,

And, always procreate the capacity to love and apply."

Borrowing 10 words from illustrious Mary K. Browne's dedication in her first book, "Top-Flite Tennis" (1928), to the game, ". . . so finely conceived is tennis that time cannot change nor custom state its infinite variety", to apply to Cissy Harris' deferential regard, marveling esteem, and daughterly love for Kurt, she writes . . .

I found a photo of Kurt with me at my house for a party - - the 100th birthday of my house.

We were great friends; we rallied together every day for many years. We would play an hour and a half late every afternoon - rain or shine.

We talked about everything that came to mind. He had such insightful comments and a rich history of almost everything. But we did not sit and talk for very long. We loved just hitting the tennis balls back and forth during our long rallies.

When we could not rally for some reason, we would read Shakespeare plays out loud at the Cal Club. We would find a quiet room and become individual characters in many of the plays.

Kurt loved food and would often greet me at the court with a "tidbit to try" . . . hummus was one of his favorites to make. He would greet his fellow friends at the Cal Club with a friendly, "How are you, Boycheck?" He would sing a loud "yahoo" if he hit a grand shot. He would often tell others to "bend their knees"! He would "thank you for sharing" when he did not feel like being interrupted or listening. And he always told me to "not forget my smile" if I was headed somewhere after tennis that I was not looking forward to doing. He would always ask me what I planned to wear.

I miss Kurt. He was kind, gentle, and good. I call his daughter Lenny every year on his birthday. He died in 2007 on his own birthday surrounded by family holding my hand.

. . . plus, a few words of her own baptism into tennis,

<u>Cissy Harris</u>

I am honored to be asked to talk about myself.

I was born and raised in San Francisco. My parents met at Stanford. My father's second-generation company manufactured garden hoses. My mother and father were both college athletes. My father played football. My mother was a skier. My two brothers and I were encouraged to have different sports. One brother played high school football and one was a boxer at Cal. I was ten when my mom suggested I "try tennis". It was "love at first stroke". I played all the time! I played public tournaments and joined the California Tennis Club as soon as it was allowed. I had to be twelve. I played for Cal, and I still play whenever I can.

I have taught 3-, 4-, and 5-year-olds for the last 35 years at the same school. When I conference with parents, I always tell them how important it is for a child to have a sport. They benefit in so many ways: peer recognition, friendship, confidence, and a sport keeps the children focused and "out of trouble". Also, it becomes a wonderful focus and passion.

Best of all - it is always fun!

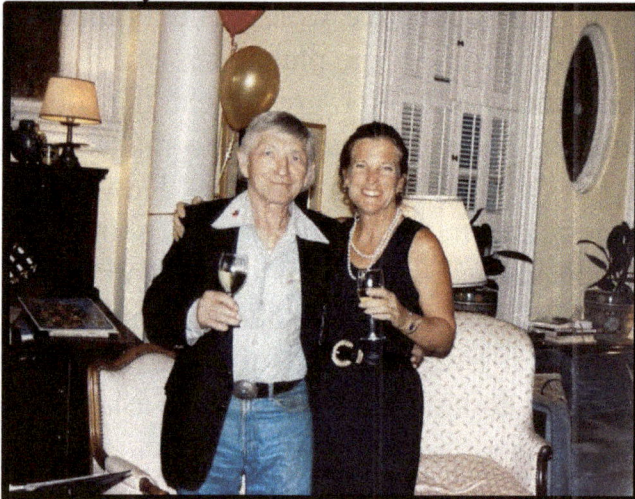

(Kurt & Cissy)

58

Gordon Readey

Member of the Pebble Beach Tennis and Swim Club, California

My love for tennis stems from three areas:

1) Builds self-reliance
2) Brings the world together
3) You can play it your whole life

#1 - There's nowhere to turn when you're down in a match, feeling fatigue, and mentally discouraged. It's hot. The sun is beating down and all of your friends and family are sitting there watching you struggle. There's nowhere to hide, no teammates to blame, no coaches to help, just you and all the voices in your head. It's in these moments that you have to dig deep inside and find that extra energy but also willing to be honest about what's not working and what needs to change. These moments are difficult, but there is no better way to learn what you're capable of and what's possible when you refuse to quit. Because at the end of the day, your opponent is just as human as you are and could easily find themselves plummeting to the same depths. It's really a matter of who believes in themselves more. Who thinks they physically have what it takes but also who has the mental skills to outsmart the other side. These self-reliance skills are developed on the tennis court but are invaluable off-court in school, work, and relationships.

#2 - There are few sports that are as globally celebrated as tennis. As a kid, it helped me learn about the world and instilled in me a sense of being a global citizen. My favorite players have been German, Czech, Spanish, Australian, and Swiss. I think that's what always struck me is the common love and respect for the game that has pervaded every corner of the globe. There's a basic civility and sportsmanship that each player brings to the court wherever they come from. To me, it always emphasized that the sport was bigger than any one individual or country. The traditional "good match" at the end of each match is the best illustration, but there are smaller gestures that are just as powerful; apologizing when your ball catches the tape and drops for a winner or checking on your opponent after they've taken a tumble on the court. Despite all the things that divide us these days, these basic displays of respect for the game help remind us what we have in common.

#3 - This one pretty much speaks for itself. I few up watching my father and his friends play every Sunday. It was heated and competitive but mainly, it was social and a way for all involved to get some good exercise. There were close calls and long rallies, but every match ended with high fives and back slapping, regardless of who carried the day. This is a game I play today into my 40s and I look forward to playing into my 50s, 60s, and beyond. While the game may become less physical, you still have the mental strategy around identifying opponents' weaknesses and practicing that self-reliance we talked about earlier.

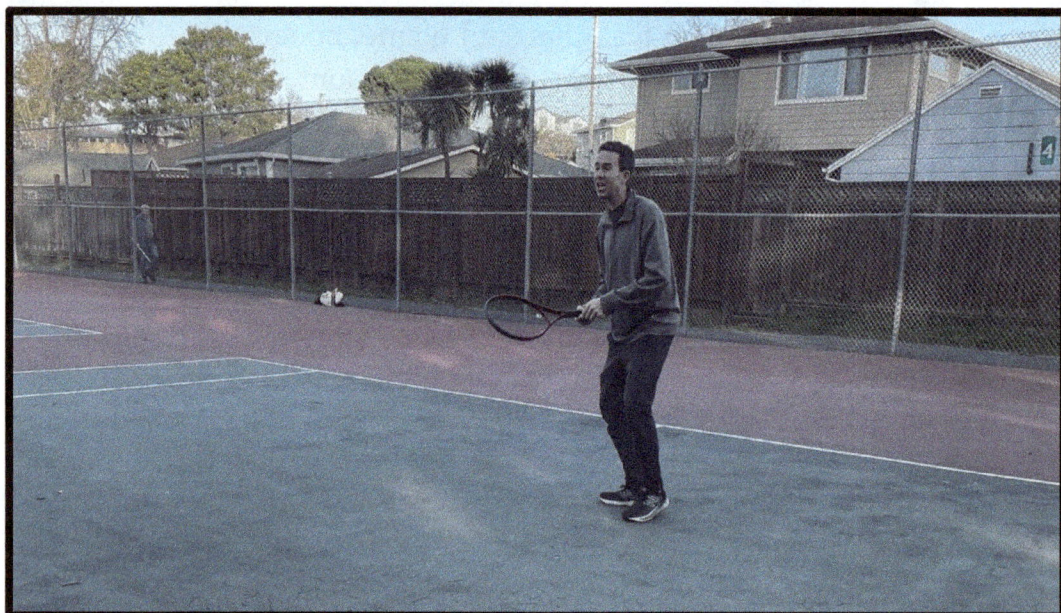

(Gordon Readey)

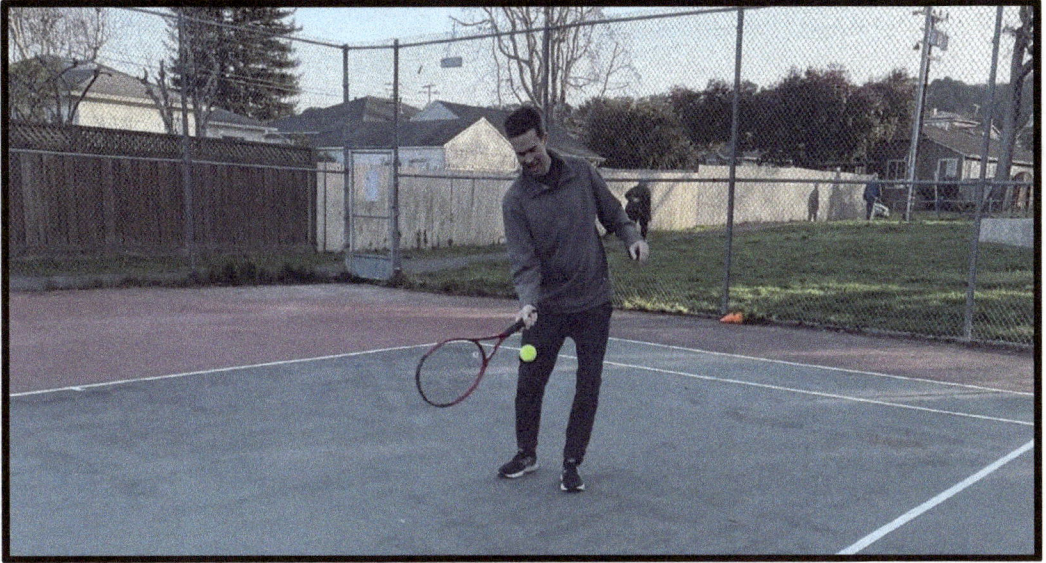

(Gordon Readey)

<u>Wendy Grover</u>

We started playing tennis at our little tennis club called Brookside in Saratoga, Ca. It was the THING to do back in 1966. And in the summer, they brought in a tennis pro and we ALL took lessons. This pro named Martin worked like a dog all day with white stuff on his lips! I remember the day he gave up trying to teach us a one-handed backhand and finally taught us the two-handed and POOF! Just like Chrissie Evert. I loved it and continue to teach it today! I got quite good and began to teach at a private court in Saratoga and then went on to play in college.

My parents loved playing and we all went to the club, played tennis all weekend. My mom signed us up for some tournaments, but the real tennis players were my two younger brothers who ended up being ranked in NorCal at eight and ten years old, and my mom drove them everywhere for lessons and tournaments. My son, Casey, learned to play with Mike Trabert at the beach club and that is when he loved it. He played on the RLS boys tennis team and taught for Steve Proulx out at Carmel Valley Tennis Camp where he attended as a camper. That is where Casey really learned to play after high school. The counselors there played Division One for their colleges or played for their country in the Davis Cup. These were phenomenal players and Casey learned so much. Then Casey taught tennis at UCLA! When my granddaughter was three, I had her on the courts for 20 to 30 minutes weekly just to get used to courts, balls, and racquets and of course etiquette and good sportsmanship. Kai is now in 8th grade, and I hope she plays for me in high school here at RLS.

Jeff Young, the AD at the time, was considering a new girls tennis coach. I was competing against all the male pros. I went to Jeff, who has two daughters, and I said that girls need a female role model, and I got the job! And have been there ever since!

My mom began our tennis lessons at Brookside Tennis Club in Saratoga one summer when I was twelve. Never looked back.

I began teaching at 17.

When I teach little ones, it is for just five minutes. At the net, two-handed backhanded volleys with the soft tennis balls. I put the balls right on their racquet and praise them endlessly. Their focus ends after a few minutes and then they want to use the tubes to pick up balls! You can have them every day for five minutes until they ask for more.

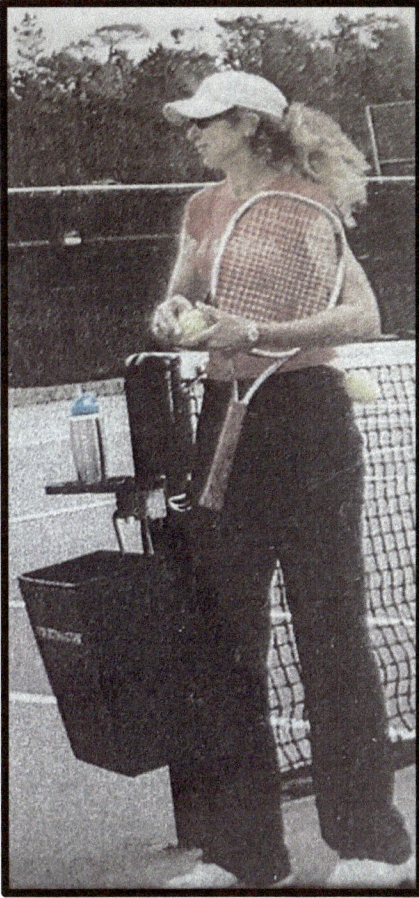

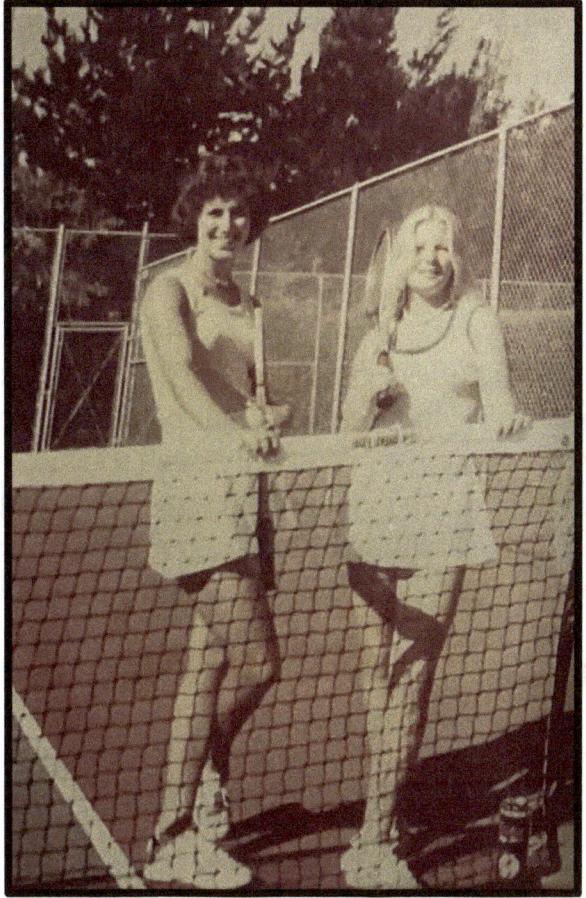

(Wendy Grover)

63

Dani Dayton

I took my first tennis lesson when I was 46 years old. Growing up, I didn't have the opportunity to play tennis. When I was in my 30's, I played tennis for the very first time when I started playing Singles with my husband. He was self-taught and gave me some "pointers." Other than that, I had no training. Along the way, I picked up some very bad habits. Then, when I was 46, I was asked to play Doubles with a women's tennis league. I jumped in, with both feet. I knew I had to up my game, so I took my very first lesson…at age 46. I am 53 now. I love the game of tennis. I still take lessons and clinics. I'm still trying to correct the years of bad habits. Trying to obtain that perfect stoke. Tennis is a game you can play your whole life. You only need to find one other person to play with. Or it could just be you hitting against a backboard or ball machine.

This is why it was extremely important to me for my two sons to take both private lessons and to enjoy fun-filled tennis camps in the Summer when they were very young. I wanted them to learn perfect form and avoid developing bad habits. I also wanted them to enjoy the journey of learning such an amazing game. I truly feel that I've given them a special gift that they can use throughout their life.

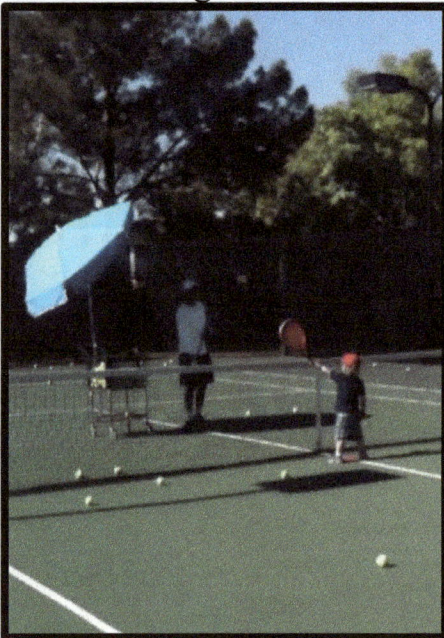

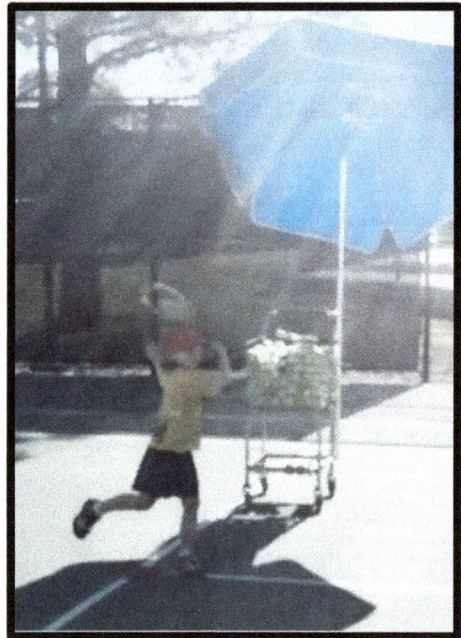

The Inspiring Legend of John Gardiner's Tennis Ranch, Carmel Valley,California

In a splendidly written article entitled "Step, Step, Step In, Hit!", which appeared in "Forest News", a Del Monte Forest Property Owners' Bulletin published in an issue dated July-September 2022, Charles Osborne, a long-standing resident of the Forest and its Pebble Beach, traces the origin, growth, and development of an awesome idea that soon became a legend. "Step, Step, Step In, Hit!" was our mantra when taking lessons from John Gardiner, the much-admired coach at the Beach and Tennis Club in the 1950s.

Charley is the grandson of Sam Morse, a legendary developer who almost singlehandedly established Pebble Beach. Sam talked John Gardiner into becoming Director of Tennis at the Beach and Tennis Club in the late 1940s. Later, John developed the Tennis Ranch in Carmel Valley which in turn spawned 10 other John Gardiner Tennis Ranches in the U.S. Among the world's top tennis players, Ken Rosewall, who assisted him in establishing a Tennis Ranch in Scottsdale, Arizona.

F⦁RESTNEWS

**Del Monte Forest
Property Owners**
a non-profit California Corporation
JULY - SEPTEMBER 2022

STEP, STEP, STEP IN, HIT! - BY CHARLES OSBORNE

Step, Step, Step in, Hit! That was our mantra when taking tennis lessons from John Gardiner, the much admired coach at the Beach and Tennis Club in the 1950's.

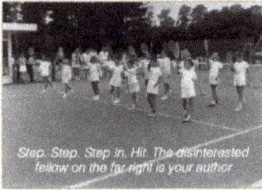

He taught us not only the game, but the etiquette and the joy of tennis. He would say, "Take your racket with you when you travel, and you will make three new friends." He would advise us, "White is always right" in tennis apparel. Try telling that to Serena Williams today. He also felt that "Repetition is the law of learning," and drilled us endlessly.

Step. Step. Step in. Hit. The disinterested fellow on the far right is your author

John was born in Philadelphia in 1918 and took up tennis at an early age. He loved the sport and was well regarded as a player and instructor. He went to Pennsylvania Teachers College, and when the war started he enlisted in the Army Air Corps. Afterwards, he moved to Monterey and coached the Monterey High School football team to their only undefeated season ever.

S. F. B. Morse, a former star football player himself, was impressed with Gardiner's success as a coach and asked him to come to Pebble Beach to be the sports director and run the tennis program. The sports director's job included running the golf tournaments like the Bing Crosby Pro-Am, the sailing regattas and the road races. This was in addition to launching and promoting a full-scale tennis operation.

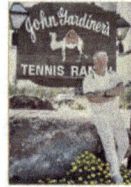

John had plenty of ideas on how to promote the tennis program in Pebble Beach. He staged exhibitions with stars like Pancho Gonzales, Tony Trabert, Jack Kramer and Ken Rosewall. He liked to note afterwards that he only paid them $1,000, and they had to make their own beds. He had his friend Clint Eastwood host a celebrity tournament. In the end however, Pebble Beach was and is a golf mecca, and John knew he needed a resort focused just on tennis to fit his plans.

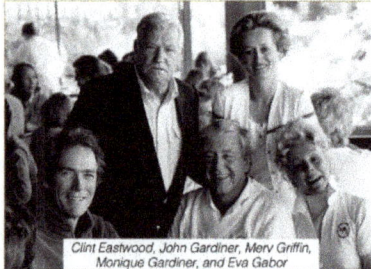

Clint Eastwood, John Gardiner, Merv Griffin, Monique Gardiner, and Eva Gabor

When a chicken ranch in Carmel Valley came up for sale, he saw it would be perfect for his plan. The place needed a lot of work to meet his ideas, and he needed financing. He shared the idea with Morse, who fired him on the spot! Morse was very loyal to his employees and expected the same from them. However, the next day Morse called him back to the office, and said he would hire him back at double the salary because "you'll need that money to start your ranch." John was able to secure financing with the help of Morse, Russ Gallaway and others.

Continued on page 2

It was here that he developed not just the kids, but also their parents, celebrities and tennis lovers. You could be playing in the court next to Clint Eastwood or John Wayne. Billie Jean King could be having a warm-up rally with Bobby Riggs while Allen Greenspan and Helen Wills Moody were playing mixed doubles with Sandra Day O'Connor and George Bush.

All of these and many more spent time at one of his ranches or clinics. Politics were not important at the tennis ranch, but it was where Ronald Reagan made his decision to run for Governor of California.

John hosted a tournament for U.S. Senators appropriately called the Senators Cup. More than 20 members joined in. Later he dedicated a wing to the Hospice of the Valley in Scottsdale where his wife died and listed on a plaque

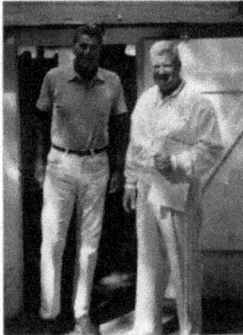

Reagan and Gardiner

all the senators and their states that had played in the tournaments, but not their political party. Tennis is non-partisan. He had such a profound influence on the sport he was elected to the Hall of Fame for the Southwest and taught thousands of people how to improve their game and enjoy it.

His brainchild, the tennis ranch, was just as it sounds. Kids would live in dormitories and play tennis at least 6 or 7 hours a day with a break for lunch. The camps lasted 3 weeks, and it was guaranteed your game would be raised several notches. I went to

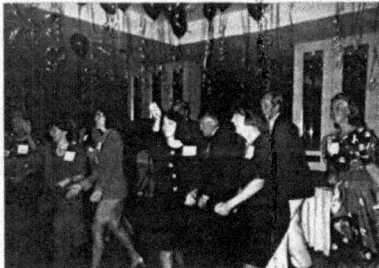

Stepping in 40 years and several cocktails later

one of the first sessions at the Tennis Ranch in 1959 and my son (now 35) went to his last in 2000. I noticed the bunks in the dorm looked exactly the same...but maybe had new mattresses. After attending the camp I found every school we played against had Tennis Ranch veterans.

Adults enjoyed it too. Their food was much better, and they could relax in their casitas or play tennis and take classes at their leisure. It was an immediate success. The casitas were booked solid as were the camps. They would have to turn away over 300 kids each year due to strong demand.

The second Tennis Ranch was in Scottsdale, Arizona and that is when his teaching methods and his tennis resorts became famous. In the end there were 11 John Gardiner Tennis Ranches and clinics in the U.S. all using John's method of instruction...repetition, footwork, grip and stroke.

Tennis became very popular in the post war era and continued with the Kennedy fitness craze. His vision of the Tennis Ranch was perfect for this. It didn't hurt that John was a very nice man, sociable, entertaining and a great story teller. His daily uniform of long cream colored pants, white Izod tennis shirt and a white wool sweater with "V" stripes stood out on the court. His black Irish hair turned pure white in time, but his smile never faded.

2

67

John was a firm believer in etiquette, dress codes and getting spoiled little rich kids off their rear ends and running around. We had to sweep and maintain the courts, collect balls and other tennis related tasks besides running tennis drills and playing competitively.

He was always nice to us. I remember a time on the courts one of the students complained that I was slow (I was), and Mr. Gardiner said "Charley may be slow, but he's quick." I loved that.

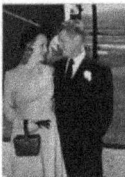
John and Barbara at the Lodge in Pebble Beach on their wedding day in 1948

John was the visionary, but it was his wife Barbara who ran the company. She was not only the business manager, but did everything from hand printing the daily menus to running the clubhouse store. All agree that without her diligence, the ranches would not have survived. The family lived on the ranch in Carmel Valley and every evening at dinner John would ask his kids, John Jr., Tom, Tricia and Tenise, "What did you do for the ranch today?"

Two years after Barbara died from a long battle with cancer in 1978, he married Monique Ledoux. Monique was well regarded for her elegant style and her gardening expertise. She allowed others to run the mechanics of the business but was the ultimate decision maker.

By the year 2000 when John died, the popularity of tennis had started to decline and the kids' programs were eliminated. The ranches were sold per the terms of John's will, but his clinical methods are carried on today anywhere tennis is taught.

Those of us who had the privilege of learning from him are very thankful for that experience. Two of his former students, Bill Stahl and Jody Bunn, hosted a reunion in 1993 where over 200 people crammed into the Beach Club dining room to celebrate him…at one point the former students got up and stood in rows in front of John as they chanted the mantra and moved in unison to " STEP, STEP, STEP-IN, HIT." ❧

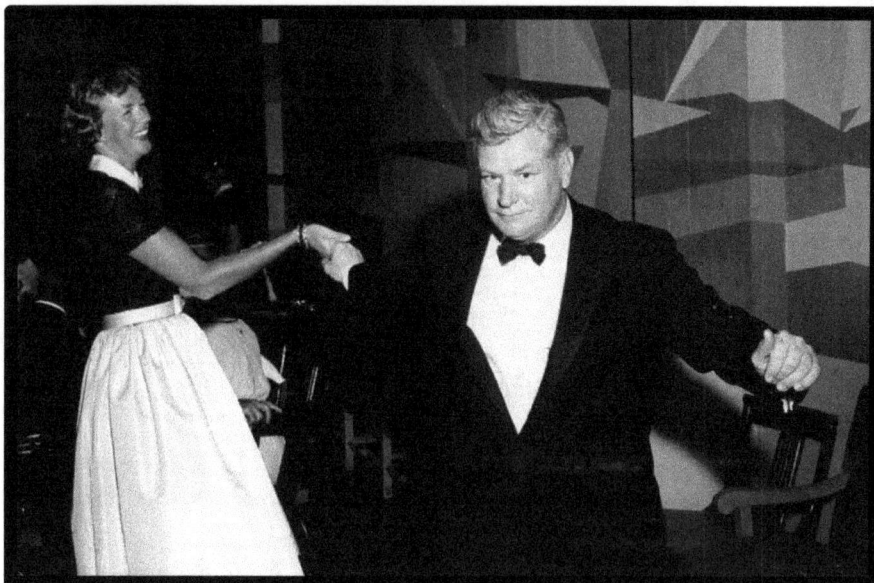

(John Gardiner)

Chapter Two

"Mommy, Daddy, will you teach me how to play tennis?"

Desirable Learnings for Toddlers
Children want to be free,
and the genuine pleasure found in tennis frees them to do so;
Believing the sport can be taught at two…

From state pre-school teachers and Head Start planners to entire elementary school faculties, and from university presidents supervising their Schools of Education Deans monitoring professors cultivating other teachers in the normal aptitudes of children for exercise, play, observation, imitation, and construction while emphasizing social training and activities, the conviction and belief continues. 90% of a child's memory, and brain has developed by the age of five, his or her past 60 months having set the curved path, or orbit, for the young life. The Jesuits of the Society of Jesus, a Roman Catholic monastic brotherhood for men founded in 1534, may have had it right, "Give me the child until he is five, and you and society can have him back for the rest of life."

If true that 90 % of the child's brain develops by age 5, we then argue that what happens in those first five years underscore how important it is to ensure his or her access to high-quality, nurturing early learning experiences that guarantee success.

Why tennis, and all schooling, should begin at two years . . .

One of the main aims of education, and tennis, is to enlighten the minds of young kids to the importance of their physical bodies, to be aware of life's dangers, to sensitize safety over risk to self and others. In short, to patiently explain, train, instruct, emphasizing to achieve for oneself understanding by doing or solving. The new medical, psychological, and educational professions know that between the ages one, two, and three growth of brain tissue accelerates, reinforcing what boys and girls learn in those three years depends on what they have become between birth and two. If free of violence, hunger, abandonment, loneliness, and excessive and cruel discipline, and sincerely and warmly wanted and respected as a natural evolving identity, "the twig has been bent", as the Jesuits have been saying for more than seven centuries, for lifelong growth and development, and for the human's ultimate goal, self-realization, the actualization of the self to help others less fortunate. Elementary education at the earliest stages, i.e., preschool, kindergarten, first grade, then second, etc., foster dormant but never forgotten lessons such as learning to control and handle one's body; how to relate to others, even if the others are despicable; engaging in healthy playful sporting activities; and becoming increasingly aware of the harmful habit patterns, some more difficult and challenging to discern than others. Happy, loved, kind, and gentle children, must, must, must understand evil is always near, but that no baby was ever born evil.

As the brain grows and expands beyond the age of two, so does curiosity and its incredible number of interests. Kids want to play and laugh, to see, hear, taste, and smell everything. By using their sense organs, they learn, developing their mind even further. What is learned may remain deeply unconscious, or perhaps at the subconscious or preconscious levels, but will never be forgotten, often surfacing six to eight or nine decades after the event. We've stated that the mental activities associated with early positive experiences lay the foundation upon which later successes in learnings, such as reading, mathematics, writing, and even sports are based. But in today's often-scattered world, it's more difficult for the home to provide all the foundational positive experiences. Since education emanating from the senses, which benefits children the most at age two to three in the home, is inundated due to a variety of family issues, a schoolyard, park, and even a tennis court can provide what the home lacks by way of special equipment, companions of the same age, and time before supper.

For centuries in our America, formal education has largely focused upon the ages between 6 and 16. Today, virtual every one of us, including our friends around the world, believes teaching should be intensified not only at the elementary level, but also in the pre-school years due to the mounting evidence that the smallest children at the tenderest ages are bestowed with the greatest gift nature can provide, other than maximum health - - the astounding massive capacity to learn from the moment after birth.

Of course, excessively loving, nurturing, and nourishing mothers who know how to step back slowly, gradually, quietly upon giving their milk have known about this positive instinct from their first moment of fondling the life they brought into the world, just as early, intuitive Cro-Magnon moms did before history. Dr. Minnie Berson, former U.S. Office of Education Coordinator, Early Childhood Programs, repeatedly argued, taught, announced, to any or all who would listen,

"There is no longer any question that the very youngest of infants are open to learning . . . after all they had to learn to survive. I am not alone in now believing that the youngest years are the most crucial of all for learning. We are dismayed when told parents and teachers underestimate the true intellectual potential of children during the preschool years. Most of the academic worlds are challenging the traditional child-rearing precepts while helping to develop more stimulating programs that accelerate the learning of the young."

In 1965, committee members of the Association for Childhood Educational International in Washington, DC, sat down with others to plan a book entitled simply as "Feelings and Learning", emphasizing the significance of emotional thought, i.e., feelings, as a neglected facet of learning today and related to children to continuous growth. The goal of that wonderful committee was to put their book in the hands of parents, hoping their children would be the ultimate benefactors. In her contributions, "Children Want to Be – Feelings About Himself and Herself Are Shaped by Feelings of Trust", "Gadgets and Feelings, Competence, Values", and "Satisfactions of Learning with Frustrations Part of Life", all three cogently reminding us that the growing-up process includes the maturing of feelings as well as the maturing of understanding and skills, and the feelings of the child have much to do with the process of development of his skills and knowledge. When he is quite young, he chooses primarily . . . . what feels good at the moment."

Lest we forget, Minnie Berson reminded, two- to three-year-old children want to be accepted, liked, respected, and "trusted friendly active inside and behind things", able to test their strength, daring, successful, able to achieve, permitted time to daydream, identify with adults who are important to them, above all, parents who are critical in their lives.

71

Independent, amused, exhilarated by rough play, involved in tasks significant to them, helpful to others, able to explore the joys of living: the dance, able to experiment with instruments,

adequate in meeting physical situations adequate in meeting intellectual situations, supported

when hurt, responsible for helping themselves, given an opportunity to explain mistakes,

encouraged in their work, free to initiate new activities, free to experiment with old materials in new ways. Simply put, children want to be themselves," she argued, insisted, taught.

As the co-authors of this Volume 1, we conclude Chapter One by a quote, one of the finest, truest, statements in the century and a half of world tennis as we know it today. It was penned in the late 1920s by Mary K. Browne, three times Champion of America, National Women's Single Champion, National Women's Doubles Champion, Captain of the Wightman Cup Team, a fine, highly intelligent, gracious, kind, gentle woman, a true "tenniser" who not only championed American leadership and supremacy, but also endeared herself spiritually to the entire Nation in those years for her humility, openness, and honesty. She wrote the following Foreword for her first book entitled "TOP-FLITE TENNIS", 1928.

Athletic Sport As A Training School For Life

"I believe there is no better way to train youngsters in the art of facing and defeating the problems of life than through the medium of athletic sports.

If they have acquired any degree of success at their game, they have learned all the essential qualities of sportsmanship and discipline which will contribute substantially to their success in business. The story of so many successful businessmen is the story of many successful athletes:

An aptitude rather than any startling genius or physical gift;

A capacity for relentless practice and hard work;

A love, without reservation or qualification, for the game played;

A focus of thought and energy;

A desire to win only outweighed by a determination to play fair."

Usually, Mary concluded her writings by citing one of her favorite hoped-for, enduring quotations, "Sportsmanship is Noble Character in its most courageous and gallant form defined: Sportsmanship (noun) is a skill in or devotion to sports, esp. conduct becoming to a sportsman, involving honest rivalry and graceful of result."

-Webster's Merriam Series New College Dictionary of the English Language, 1956.

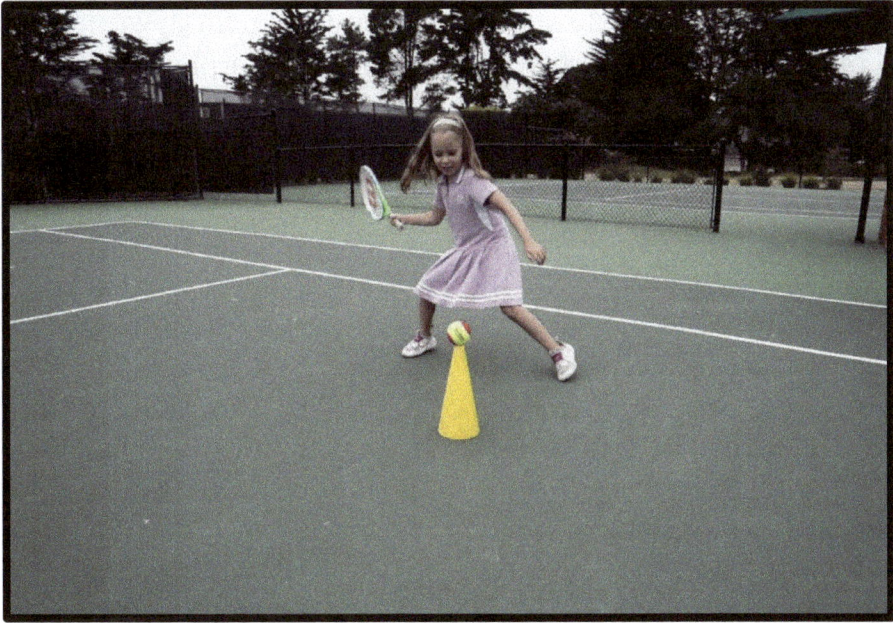

Two self-understanding, self-improving questionnaires about child growth and development

Since the 1920s, psychologists, educators, philosophers, scientist and mathematicians, even popular actors and athletes, have formulated elementary, imperfectly developed, vestigial thoughts and "theories" on how children learn best - - mostly by observing the educational successes of their own children. We must never forget that kids construct their own images of the world, family, and people from their experiences of them in their own stimulating or unstimulating environmental world. Like our faithful mentors, Mary K. Browne, Lois Barclay Murphy, Mercer Beasley, etc., we, too, confirm the extraordinary importance of a child's growing process in the first several years of life.

Evolving psychology, the study of the growth of intellect in children and how its various attributes blossom, had a great influence on parental beliefs in the early 1920s. The early educators trusted the theories of Jean Piaget, the renowned Swiss psychologist who formulated a new understanding of child growth and development by studying his own three kids. Another theorist American educators and parents idolized Germany's Friedrich Frobel who in the early 19th Century not only created the concept of the "kindergarten", but also coined its term while developing educational toys known as "Frobel Gifts".

Soon, across America, college educated, intellectually sophisticated women, especially mothers with young children, were particularly entranced by the Frobel learning-toys, smooth Maplewood rectangles, squares, cube, cylinders, brightly colored odd-shaped blocks, i.e. tassels, shiny paper, long cylindrical rods to buttress whatever creations emanated from the young elastic imaginations. Such fiercely independent mothers idolized their boys, many of whom became famous i.e., Winston Churchill, John D. Rockefeller, Douglas MacArthur, Ulysses Simpson Grant, and countless others. Because such moms did not trust local teachers to properly educate their own flesh and blood, they simply taught their boys and girls themselves. One mother, Anna Lloyd-Jones was determined, without reservation or qualification, to shape son, Frank Lloyd Wright, into the greatest architect who ever lived. In her pregnancy, she dreamed and determined, then determined and dreamed. Right after his birth, she posted ten full-page wood-engravings of old English cathedrals around his crib-to-be. Above the crib were brightly colored thin mobiles set in motion by air currents. Many of the magazine photos of historic world structures were framed. All educators, then and now, clearly see the point: a mom's tender fervor lovingly expressed patiently can indeed work miracles!

Before proceeding, try a true or false question, written by Dr. Joyce Brothers based on experts' opinions for her San Francisco Examiner page 10 column on September 9th, 1978. Although judgements and convictions held firmly at the time, the authors of this text are of the sentiment the answers are grounded in truth, even approaching a half a century later.

1. If a little girl, especially a 1-year-old, wants to be adven-turous, her parents should hold her back.

FALSE. Psychologist Louise Kaplan has observed that from 10-15 months, the child is a high-spirited conqueror hero, exploring and manipulating the world around him or her. This is when mothers damage daughters out of a mistaken notion that girls are more fragile than boys. If a girl is encouraged to cling, the being-done-to element in her personality isn't sufficiently balanced by the sense of mastery and active doing-to.

2. Three-and-4-year-olds should get used to being away from their parents.

TRUE. This helps them to learn to be more independent. It also prepares them for the first time they must leave the parents to go to school.

3. If parents prepare and teach a child as much as possible before he starts school, he will do well in the first few years and be happier.

FALSE. According to psychologist Dr. Lovick Miller elaborate preparations at home may make him anxious. It also won't help the child's learning because teachers have standard format and the system parents use may prove to be all wrong.

4. Children are never depressed or suicidal.

FALSE. Children suffer from periods of depression in much the same way adults do. A recent study of more than 1,000 children aged 6 to 17 who were treated at poison control centers revealed that 74 percent of the cases were either genuine suicide attempts or suicide gestures -- attempts made with the knowledge that they will not succeed.

5. The "peek-a-boo" game is an important learning tool.

TRUE. Peek-a-boo is one of the earliest interpersonal communications. It not only establishes a way of responding to overtures, but also establishes self-confidence and an early sense of identity.

6. Girls are more apt to have a bed-wetting problem than boys are.

FALSE. Four out of five cases of bed-wetting occur in boys. Some go on wetting fairly steadily till 6, 8, 10 or even 12 years of age.

7. Discipline and punishment are basically the same thing.

FALSE. Discipline limits behavior and provides guidelines. Punishment is the result of violating discipline. Punishment should be meted out by withdrawal of privileges rather than by physical punishment.

8. Motherhood is almost always a joy and a blessing from the newborn's very beginning of life.

FALSE. This isn't true and because some women have unrealistic expectations about the "joys" of motherhood, they may blame the child when these expectations are not fulfilled. Dr. Bertram Cohler, a Chicago psychologist, says that next to a death in the family, often, the most stressful event in a woman's life is giving birth.

In continuing your self-awareness questionnaire, please resharpen your pencil and take another moment to engage in a second 8-question "Agree" or "Disagree" pop quiz from the Foreman-DeNevi Tenants of Winning Tennis Test regarding parental love, physical growth and generation, and development of psychological health in their child.

1. In addition to years of playing the game, tennis can be life-changing and lifesaving, and wonderful fun at the same time.

2. Displaying effusive elation by mom, dad, and family seeing their child eagerly learning and playing the game will not only intensify the expectation to continue, but the education of it will heighten his or her IQ level significantly.

3. The attention, approval, and affection a mother and father give their child are all extremely powerful reinforcements. For example, a

baby can be taught to lift its arm when a lamp is turned off and on. If and when a baby does something successful, he should be rewarded with parental cheers to try other new movements.

4. The creation of a national program of early childhood education reaching every youngster in the country starting at age two or two-and-a-half should be initiated immediately substantiating the continued growth of evidence that a high portion of intelligence is clearly and permanently shaped before a child enters kindergarten at age five.

5. Between ages two and three, growth of brain tissue takes place, and what children learn in that year is carried over into later life. Learning to handle their bodies, to relate to others, to become aware of the meanings of things about them are all basic learnings. Between ages two and three, many new habit patterns are formed, so the child's education during that year is important. There is no reason why tennis and other sports shouldn't be introduced along with other recreational sports, and arts and crafts.

6. In short, the first child's impressions and lessons are never forgotten.

7. Tennis nurtures emulation, poise, calmness, character, lasting curiosity, physical fitness, honesty, self-consciousness, emotional health and confidence, joy in action, culture awareness, the arts and humanities, in short, all that is good for the natural growth and development of the child, among a host of his or her fledgling interests.

8. Two and three-year-olds, like kindergarteners two years later, pull information from the people and environments around them. They want to know everything, i.e., who cuts their hair, examines and pulls teeth, writes the newspapers, repairs shoes, pilots airplanes, enforces laws, delivers mail, takes care of the forests, etc, etc. Soon, hopefully, attention will focus upon tennis, whose success is determined by the curiosity about the life it fosters.

Tom Moore
Tennis Instructor

Junior Summer Tennis Camps Start
This Month!!

"My theory is simple. If you buy an ice cream cone and make it hit your mouth, you can learn to play tennis. If, on the other hand, the ice cream hits your forehead, your chances aren't as good . . ."

--Vic Braden, tennis instructor

Tennis isn't all about winning

"The worst thing is to do this to win. Even when I don't win, I have a heck of a time out there. The thrill of playing is what it should be about. And improving your game by mentally focusing. Enjoy it and fight like a tiger, but don't let losing bother you."

- Gardnar Mulloy (82-year-old tennis player, winner of 108 USTA Championships)

"Keep your mind clean and orderly; Likewise, will your environment and life will be clean and orderly. Can perfection be attained? Try! The young student needs to have . . . an awareness of oneself, an awareness of the world. And awareness that the world and self often do not match . . . Be philosophic, intelligent, emotional. Be artistic!"

-William T. Tilden, "The Art of Lawn Tennis," 1921

Chapter Three

Tennis starts BEFORE stepping on the court

Playing tennis actually begins before walking onto the court. Developing the hand eye coordination of a 2- or 3-year-old is key to having a positive experience with tennis. This is important because once a racquet gets involved the degree of difficulty has just quadrupled. Having the base element of developing the hand eye coordination cannot be stressed enough.

Start with blowing up a balloon and bumping the balloon in the air to keep it from hitting the ground. This exercise develops eye contact (needed for tennis) spacial awareness (judging how close you need to be to the balloon) and having fun! Have you ever seen a child not laughing when bumping up a balloon in the air? Fun and Effective, this is a recipe for success! Once bumping the balloon up in the air becomes easy try alternating between you and your young player. Count how many in a row you can bump up.

Next up is developing a catch/toss mindset. When we go to the court for the first time catching a ball is very much like receiving a ball from your opponent and the toss is linked to sending the ball back over the net. The perfect starting point with a young player is to sit on the ground and play a game called, "Rollie/Pollie". Rollie/Pollie is where you roll the ball on the ground to your young player. They in turn catch the ball and roll it back to you. You can count the number of times that are successful and see if you can match that number each time you play Rollie/Pollie. Once that becomes easy, progress to letting the ball bounce on the ground one time before you catch it. Return the ball with a soft bounce before catching it. Eyes and brain are now engaged with calibrating the bounce. Our hands now need to be re-positioned for different bounces, very much like when we are trying to hit a ball with different speeds and depth when on the court. Successful? Try standing and bouncing a ball one time with a catch between both of you. Now try moving back a little further from one another with a gentle toss and bounce before catching the ball. Each move is a progressive action that leads us to getting closer to actual success on the tennis court.

Notice both games are fun, successful, and develops the physical attributes that will be needed when going to the court. Tennis is not an easy game - the better the development of hand eye and spacial awareness the higher success rate you will have when you do make it to the court.

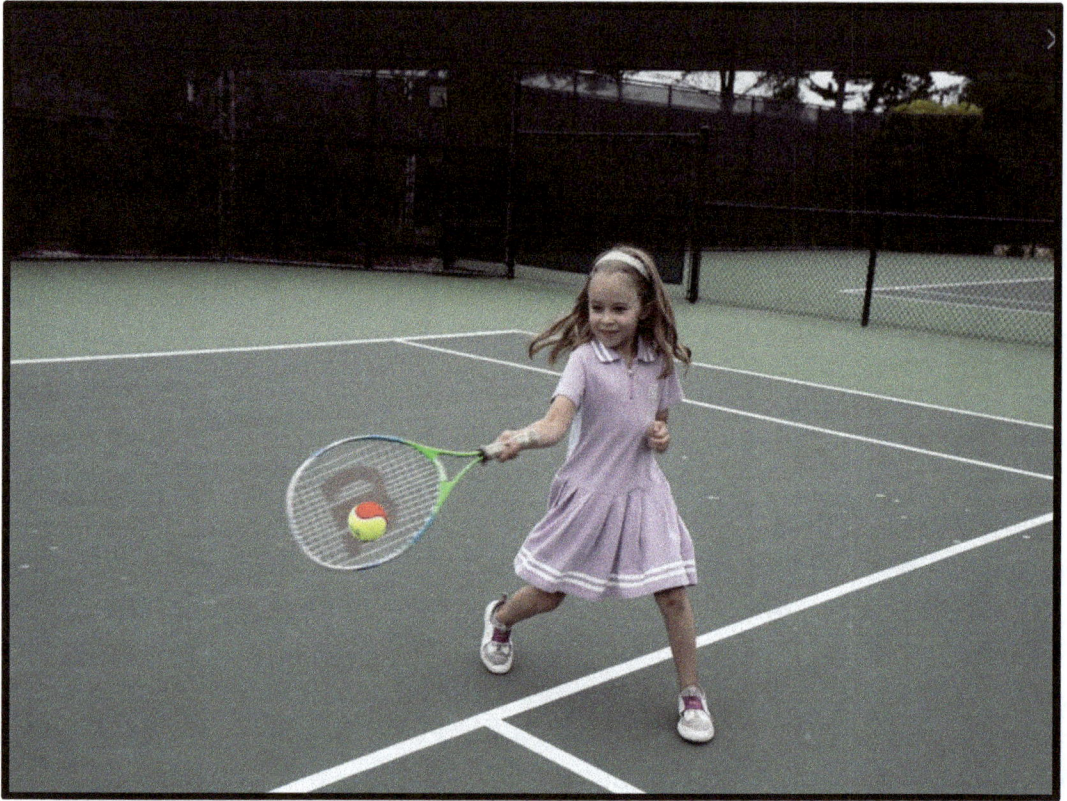

(The picture here shows the importance of the contact point. If contact on the ball with the forehand stroke is out in front. The entire body is working with the hit and maximum pace and control is optimized.)

*(Agility and movements are two elements that can be developed early!
Here we have Juliet weaving in between cones. Not only is it good for
our balance and coordination- but it's fun!)*

Chapter Four

Finding the proper racquet size and balls

Using the proper racquet size and using the correct balls are important because this will enable young players to swing at balls with a racquet that is the appropriate length and weight for better tennis, this leads to better technique and control of the racquet. Junior racquets are based on the measurement of racquet length. Junior racquets will start at 17 inches long and go to 26 inches in length (an adult frame is 27 inches). There are 2 specifications one should look at when choosing a racquet. First is age and the second is height of the player. See the table below for a guideline of racquet sizes linked to the proper age.

Ages 2 & 3 = a size 17-inch racquet.

Ages 4 & 5 = a size 19-inch racquet.

Ages 5 & 6 = a size 21-inch racquet.

The actual height of a player will also play a role in the racquet size. Sometimes a 4-year-old might be tall and have longer arm which would need a longer racquet length. So with height comes some racquet size adjustments. See table below.

Under 3 feet = 17-inch racquet.

3 feet to 3 feet 6 inches = 19-inch racquet.

3 feet 7 inches to 3 feet 10 inches = 21-inch racquet.

3 feet 11 inches to 4 feet 5 inches = 23-inch racquet.

The next important piece of equipment is using the correct tennis balls. Young players need a lower bouncing ball due to their height of their contact point. Most of the major equipment manufactures make a ball labeled as a "Red Ball". Red Balls should be used by players under the age of six. A Red Ball is larger, moves slower, and bounces lower making the ball a much easier target to hit. Success on the court at this age is all about hitting the ball over the net. With success comes the drive to get better. If our younger players are not successful, the inner drive to play diminishes and then the game becomes less fun. The secret is Success + Fun = Improvement.

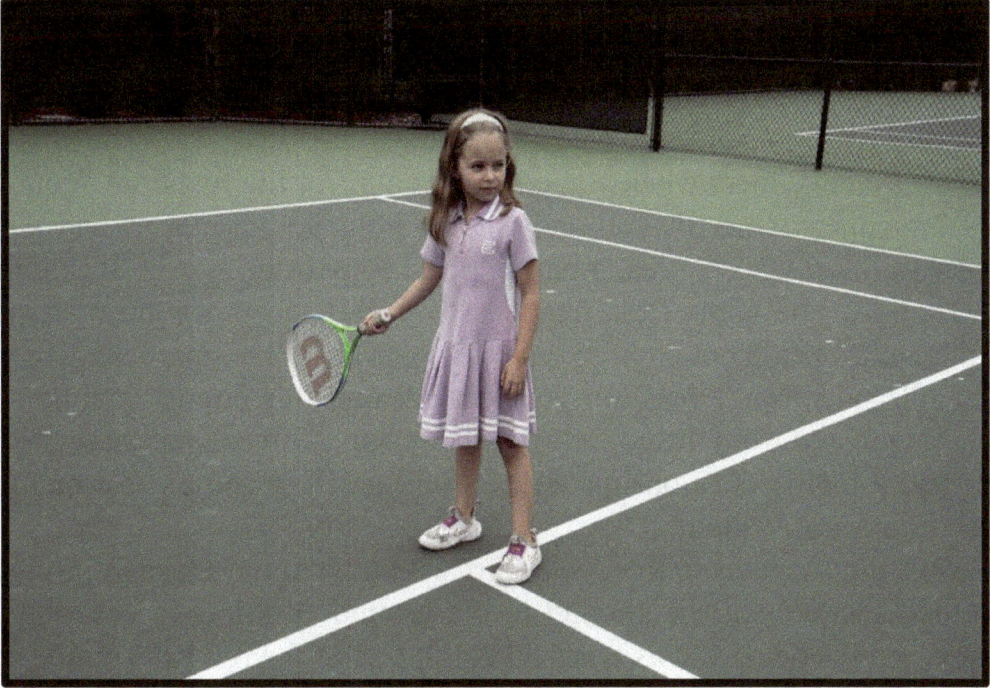

(Here Juliet is showing the importance of starting your swing with a low racquet take-back. By dropping the racquet head, it gives the lift (or clearance) of the ball over the net. Ultimately, this delivers a deep ball to your opponent.)

Chapter Five

Taking the game to the court

Here's what expect when you go to the court for the first time. You will need 2 racquets. One for you and one for your young player, and a ball hopper of "Red Balls". Yes, a ball hopper! Repetition is key. If you take three balls to the court (this happens to often) too much time is spent picking balls up and not enough time hitting. The ball hopper will give you 75 to 100 balls. Make room in your car because this hopper will be with you going to and from the court for each session. You can purchase the red balls and a ball hopper on-line. Repetition develops the muscle memory needed for improvement.

Every time you go to the court start with a warmup. Have your player turn their racquet so it is parallel to the ground. You might describe the racquet face as being flat as a pancake. Put one of the red balls on the face and walk along the lines of the court without the ball falling off the racquet. A fun game is to call out the line you are walking on. Like Baseline, doubles sideline, center service line. You are teaching your player the boundaries of the court. After you have done this a couple of times have them lead and see if they can try to remember the line's name as they walk along holding the ball on their racquet face. Remember to correct them with the proper name if a line is mistakenly called wrong. See diagram of the court and the proper boundary lines.

For the next warm-up, go the middle of the court near the service line and start dribbling the ball from the racquet to the court. This is called practicing "downs". See how many in a row you can hit. You can attempt this multiple times. Next practice "ups" this is where you are attempting to hit the ball up in the air without it touching the ground. It's a bit more difficult and the numbers of successful hits might be a lower number. Remind your young player if the racquet is held even or flat with the court the ball bouncing off the strings will be easier to control.

Chapter Six

Where to stand when feeding or tossing balls

Beginning players need a ball that bounces and can be hit at waist level. This is not as easy as it may seem. I like starting with a ball that is being tossed this helps slow down the feed and makes the contact easier for young players. You can even start tossing balls on the same side of the net as your player and this will give them a consistent contact point and a higher success rate of getting a ball over the net. You can give verbal clues while making contact with the ball. I have always liked the rhythm that is produced when a player says out loud when a ball hits the ground, "Bounce" and at the same time when they are hitting the ball, "Hit". This seems to heighten the sense of focus when ball is approaching them for a better contact point. It will also allow the player to exhale by saying the word hit, making it impossible to hold their breathe while hitting. A habit that many adult players have a hard time breaking.

Keep in mind, trying to hit a ball over the net can be a frustrating time for young players. Making contact with the ball is not easy. I like the approach of lifting the ball high so it clears the net. For now, if a ball is long or wide it is considered a good shot if it goes over the net! Again, success is the goal, which leads to fun, which is followed by improvement. As a player improves, we will be attempting to keep balls inside the lines but that's a goal saved for later tennis sessions.

Find the balance for MI. MI stands for maximum Improvement. Maximum Improvement is met when a player gets to the court for 3 sessions of tennis each week. Once a week is fine, twice a week is good, but 3 times a week is the magic number. Of course, if you get on the court more that 3 times it will show with an increase in tennis skills, timing, and ball contact. MI needs to be talked about on a regular basis. Lower court time equates to a slower improvement with the game.

<u>Chapter Seven</u>

Tennis instruction for beginners

From your toes to your nose . . . .
Bug squash . . .
Kiss your shoulder on your follow through . . .
Broken stop sign with volleys . . .
Slice the cake, serve the cake, swat the fly . . .

Young players remember phrases that stand out. These phrases will help remind us on body positioning until our muscle memory takes over. I'm going to give you some phrases so you can picture the positioning needed for success with getting the ball over the net.

From your Toes to your Nose - getting players to drop their racquet head below the ball is a challenge. When hitting a baseball, the bat rests on you shoulder. Not the case in tennis. The reference is pushing your racquet head toward to your toes on the backswing and following through over your shoulder so the racquet is finishing up by your nose. This promotes a full swing in the correct position.

Bug Squash - when a player swings their racquet it can often cause the body to become off balance. To stop any off-balance swings from taking place keep you back leg on the ground specially the toe and continue to finish up with your follow through. Your toe touching the court is very much like squashing a bug. Kids remember this one and will often remind me of the bug squash.

Kiss your Shoulder on your Follow Through - after hitting either a forehand or a two- handed backhand your follow through should bring your shoulder though the contact area to finish with your nose/mouth very close to your shoulder. Say good job and give it a quick kiss. Promotes a follow through that completes the shot and gives you a positive comment at the end.

Broken Stop Sign with Volleys - when at the net a common volley mistake is to have the racquet positioned at a 90-degree angle (straight up). You actually want the racquet head to be at a 45-degree angle. This looks like a broken stop sign. The stop sign element also reinforces the player to stop the racquet head on contact when volleying both forehands and backhands.

Slice the Cake, Serve the Cake, and Swat the Fly - serving has a multitude of things going on. It best to keep it simple - start the serve with a slicing motion with your racquet, on the downward swing. This followed by taking the racquet back by your head like to you are holding a serving tray, which then leads to swatting the fly up over your head as the racquet accelerates up for the contact on the ball.

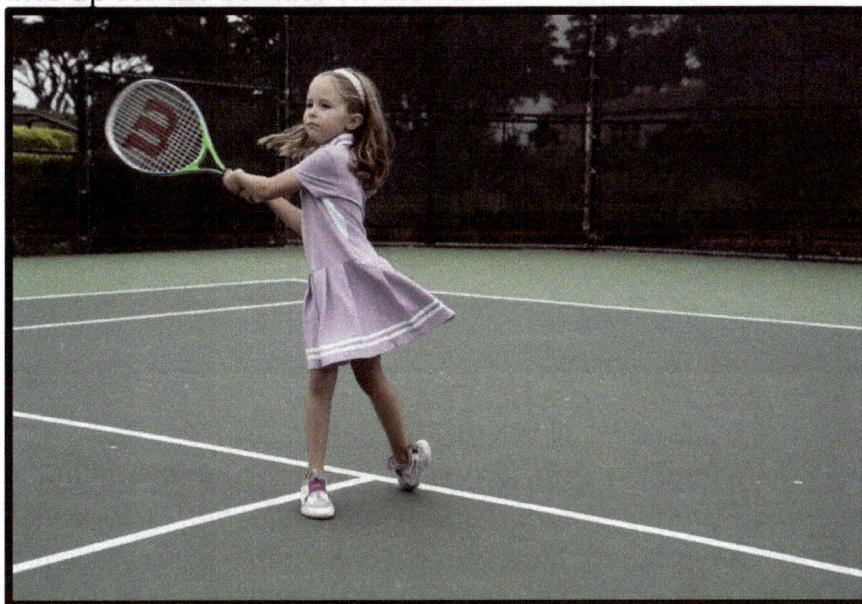

The classic "Bug Squash" follow through

(Notice Juliet's back foot? Coming up on her toe but keeping her foot on the ground behind her is giving her a balance point that will enable her to recover for the next ball quickly. This also stops the shoulders and hips from opening too soon during the contact with the ball. Kids always remember the "Bug Squash" follow through and take great pleasure in showing me their fancy footwork.)

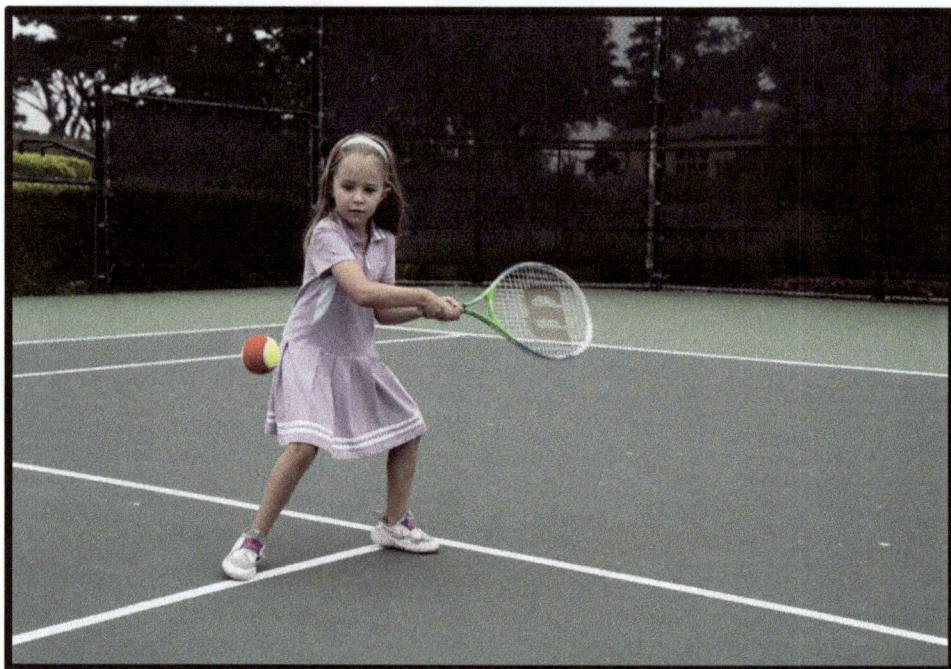

Eyes on the ball!

(Focus and seeing the ball into your racquet's strings is much easier said than done. Practice watching the seams of the ball so closely that you are able to see the direction they are moving. Using red balls helps the eye track the ball much easier for an important training tool as players get older. This is helpful when balls are being hit harder and faster as they get older.)

Chapter Eight

Developing agility and movement for better play

Importance of court ladders, cones, and circles, and jump ropes

Having the ability to move quickly on the court is a tremendous attribute to one's game and ultimately their success on the court. This is why it is so important and well worth the time to work on speed, agility, and quickness. Young players love to move and run. By taking that energy that our young players already have and structuring it in a manner that's going to pay dividends down the road. Here are some ways that will create agility, quickness, and fun!

Court Ladder - Have your players place a court ladder on the ground and have their feet step in each empty square on the ladder. It can be done by hoping on one foot in the openings of the ladder. The next time through alternate your feet so both legs are touching the ground quickly and you are "high stepping" through the ladder. Finally, the follow-up would be to step quickly to your right with your right foot leading, left foot follows closely behind, then step to the left with your left foot leading and the right foot follows closely behind. These foot work drills will showcase the importance of small steps needed to adjust quickly when a ball is hit to the forehand and then a quick adjustment for a backhand groundstroke. These drills might be difficult for younger players. You can equate the ladder to a game of hopscotch. Where you're bouncing on two feet and then to one and then back to two feet. Simon Says - can be done using the ladder with your player mimicking your steps first.

Cones & Circles - Set up 2 cones and 1 circle. The cones will have players showing their speed and coordination by running quickly in a figure 8 pattern. When using the circles, you start with both feet in the middle and then place one foot outside the circle while the other footsteps outside the circle, quickly take the foot that stepped outside the circle and move it to the inside, the remaining foot then steps inside the circle now both feet are together. Do it again leading with the other foot. This exercise is on focus and concentration. Each movement drill will last 10 seconds. You can keep a record of how many times you went around the cones or stepped inside/outside the circle. It takes time and repetition but watch how quickly players will pick up on the different maneuvers. A true test on focus, concentration, and determination. If players are having a hard time following the movement, you can easily adjust to both feet bouncing in and out of the circle using the 10 seconds as a timer to count results.

Jump Rope - One of the great exercises that has been around for a long time! When jumping rope, you are experiencing timing, foot work, breathing, and hand-eye coordination all at the same time! It can be implemented at the beginning of a tennis session as part of the warmup, or at the end before you pick up the balls before heading home.

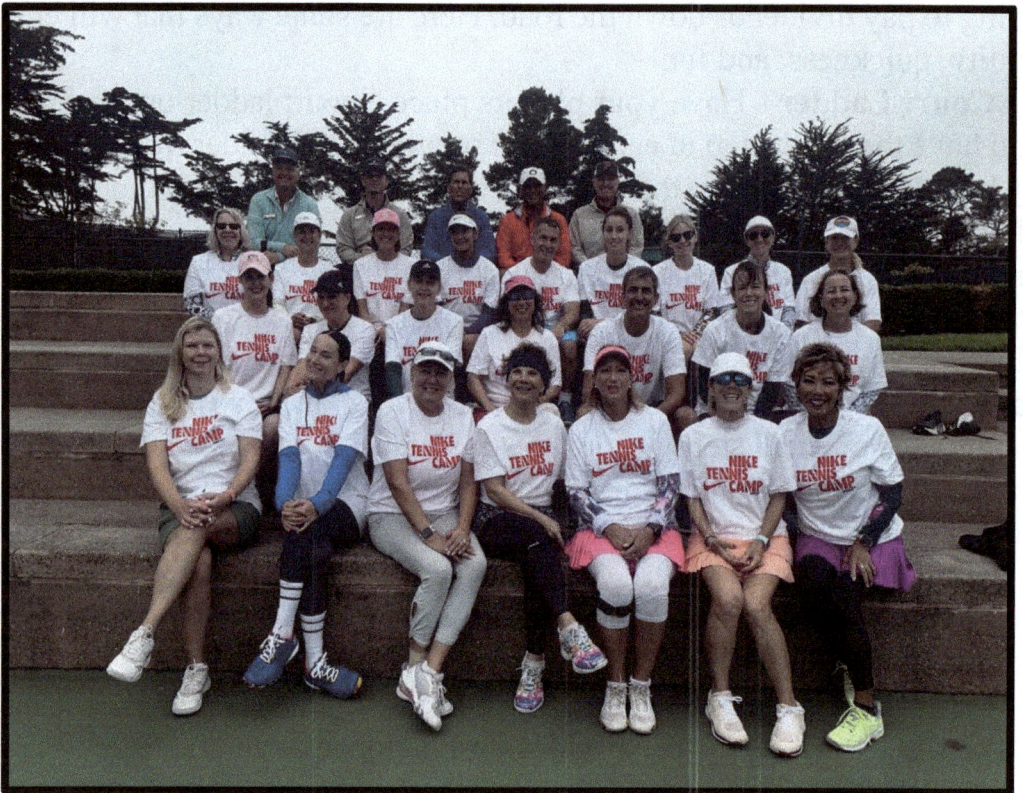

(2024 Nike Tennis Camp)

Chapter Nine

Parents Wear Many Hats

- As a parent, mother, father, family member, or even a friend, we all play an incredibly important role by forming a positive attitude with our young player. This singlehandedly is going to accelerate each achievement we accomplish.

- Make it FUN each time a racquet is picked up: With fun comes the inner drive to spend countless hours doing something we enjoy. These many hours of successful court time are filled without even realizing it! All done because of the FUN factor.

- Our young players look up to us. We need to show them how important it is to try hard, listen, be respectful, and above all things – be fair!

- Instill effort. Effort is accomplished by giving your very best every time you are on the court. By putting your best effort forward this will translate into success and the satisfaction that you did the best that you could do.

- Encourage the art of listening. This simple act of listening will help with a deeper understanding of the task at hand, it will also help with instruction, and provide an opportunity to ask questions.

- It's important your player learns to be respectful. Respect your opponent, respect the game, your equipment, and coaches. This will make your player a standout and become a natural Coaches Choice with this ability.

- Acknowledge and emphasize being fair. Tennis is a game based on fairness. Eventually your player will make their own line calls, keep track of score, and encounter situations that being fair will rise above winning or losing. Establishing the boundaries of being fair will carry your young player through the ups and downs of life as well as the ups and downs of their time when on the court.

• All of these values add up to being successful on the court. The hidden gem is the success will not only stop on the court but also become evident when faced with the many lifelong decisions that shape us into who we will become. Let's head to the court!

• Think back to a time when you were asked by a child or grandchild, "Let's go play tennis". The idea of teaching a young player a new skill might seem like a daunting task. A task that you may know very little about, or maybe it's been done, but it was a long time ago, or possibly you have never done it at all! After reading this book, your reply will be, "Yes! Grab your racquet and let's go play tennis!"

Lessons learned on the court turn into successful lifelong lessons
Keep in mind that a successful tennis player not only experiences positive results on the court, but also learns a lot about themselves that will be called upon in many different occasions. Tennis can be a frustrating sport and there is a reason it is called a game of errors. Having a successful player means they are able to understand mistakes and take action to prevent that error from repeatedly taking place.

Players make their own line calls – the honor system is tested repeatedly. How a player handles calls that go against them is not an easy task. Putting the emotions in check during a heated match is a true test that will play out in the future with business decisions, friendships, and personal relationships.

Time Management, a young player needs to prioritize between school, practice time, match play, and homework. Not easy, but again a great training ground for future situations.

Tennis is a lifetime sport. Studies have shown that by playing tennis a person extends their life by almost 10 years! In order for young players to develop a love for the game it needs to be presented in a way that a player finds a way to succeed. This is done with a successful start. Once a player finds success, the building blocks for future development are underway.

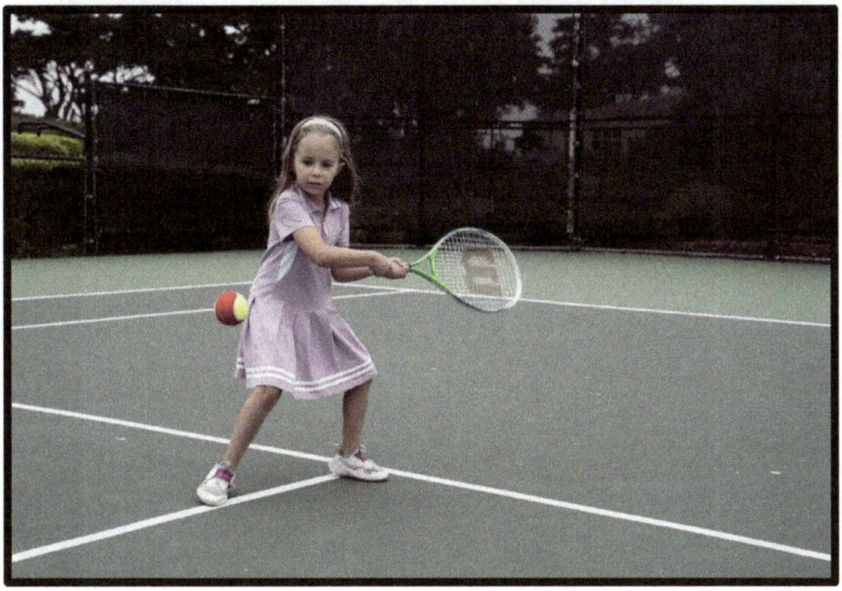

"For the child it must be today, now . . . Many other things we need can wait. The little one cannot. Right now, is the time his or her bones are being formed, his or her blood is being made, and his senses are being developed. To the child, we cannot answer 'Tomorrow'. His or her name is spelled T O D A Y !"

Gabriella Mistral, Chilean winner of the Nobel Prize for Poetry

"Education means that the student, even the youngest of the young must be drawn out of the self into other paths . . .This can only be achieved by an educative will . . . No amount of explaining can make the crooked plant grow straight; it must be trained upon the trellis of the norm by the gardener's art . . ."

Carl Jung

"Always, ever so tenderly, strive toward excellence through critical thinking. Through critical thinking we are achieving excellence, and while we are about it, on the court or at home on the living room floor, we can engage excellence by thinking critically. Back on the court, tennis provides a means to control our game, and, in looking forward, our destiny . . ."

Kurt Schlesinger, M.D, to his court friends, July 9, 1984, California Tennis Club, San Francisco

Conclusion

by Gerard Issvoran

There are many reasons to consider tennis as an initial sport for our active 2-year-old. As described earlier in the course of any particular day, there are moments for active play, which can be all-encompassing and beneficial for child development. At this point of development, we do not have to worry about rules as much as we can focus our attention on certain concepts of trying to control a tennis ball with the racquet. But even more basic than that is simply developing skills of agility which will lend themselves to any sport. Most importantly, it has to be entertaining and fun. The skills to improve agility at an early age can have long-term effects on the body for the rest of one's life. In many Eastern European countries younger children who entered tennis academies, do not even pick up a tennis racquet until they are 3 or 4 years into a program.

Group sports in this country, such as football, basketball, baseball, soccer, and hockey lend themselves to individual achievement, but it is within the context of representing their team. These team sports can play an important role in social development for any child as they learn how to play fair, support their teammates, all the while trying to improve themselves and appreciate their success.

While tennis is taught in a group setting very commonly, ultimately it is an individual sport, which lends itself to not only a greater amount of accountability but also unlocking great potential for growth and development. Down the road beyond age of 2, when winning becomes significant for an athlete in the other sports, handling success and failure takes on a different perspective. This may or may not produce the same sense in the individual world tennis or golf.

Truly, what do we remember about ourselves at age 2? In this age of advanced media. We may have videos seeing ourselves doing things that are repeated over time to ingrain a memory. But memory is affected by all of our senses, such as olfaction (smell) as well as by images that were formed early in life. What if that image was of a soft fuzzy optic yellow ball that was held in the hand and thrown, caught, or hit? Or what if that image was of being on a court with a net that was taller than your height?

95

What do we remember of the first time we were able to hit a tennis ball over the net? If these were positive experiences of running around and playing in this environment, it may have very well lent itself towards a love for a game that lasted for a lifetime.

With every sport that I have mentioned. There are graceful movements which lend themselves to a certain amount of beauty, which anyone can appreciate even if they don't understand sport. Sometimes it is the combination of power, intensity and grace which stand out even more so. The charms of a rugby scrum (not to take anything away from rugby) don't quite do it for me as much as a Roger Federer backhand, or a Pete Sampras serve. Their expression of those motions, in their tennis game were the result of that Latin phrase that I used in the forward. Along the way, the mindset of the aforementioned champions, in tennis didn't just learn tennis, rather, their ability to think, develop character, handle adversity within the context of a tennis match developed over their lifetime as they became heroic in their abilities. Understandably, very few achieve a professional level of success. Success in tennis doesn't have to necessarily do with the result as much as it is about the journey along the way. There are consequences to playing high impact sports as much as there are consequences to the long-term effects of tennis on the body. Tennis is associated with longevity.

Similar to the "rules" of the daily routines of life, tennis has lent itself as a wonderful microcosm regarding these rules of engagement which can allow us to see ourselves improve, express our way of understanding this great game, appreciate the civility of others and shake hands at the end of a match in order to say, let's do it again!

Tennis from the ground up is a concept that supports the idea that, as in most sports, unless there is a firm foundation from which a motion is generated, regardless the sport, it must be sound, strong and most importantly healthy. The beginning point for tennis, for example, must begin with the lower extremities and all of its components. As we appreciate the kinetic chain of events responsible for motion starting with the legs, we can then more fully understand how the rest of the body is affected. The goal, with identifying and understanding the various injuries that can occur throughout the body, is to help prevent, by early detection, when something goes wrong so that a serious injury can be avoided.

Because there is no aspect of the physical part of tennis that will not require some part of your body through practice or a match, we will explore the sources of pain which occur from repetitive use which involve the lower extremities, pelvis, back, neck, head, shoulders, and the rest of the upper extremities.

Ultimately, we don't want to play in fear of an injury which can trigger a sympathetic nervous system response also known as, "fight or flight". Rather, if we can perform in a state of being relaxed and not anxious, we can be at our best form to maximize and enjoy our abilities.

I will give you a little background which I hope helps for publishing purposes. I was born and raised here on the Monterey Peninsula with my big move in life at age 7 from Monterey to Pacific Grove where I attended public schools for my education. I graduated from Pacific Grove HS in 1983 and went to UC Riverside for 1 year before returning and transferring to St. Mary's College of California and receiving a Bachelor of Science as Biology/Chemistry Major focusing on molecular biology and a minor in Philosophy. I then went on to perform research in Microbiology at Cal State University, Hayward and received Post Baccalaureate Certification in Biotechnology. Thereafter, I started my medical career upon acceptance to Nova Southeastern University, College of Osteopathic Medicine in N. Miami Beach, Florida. Being homesick for California, I was accepted in one of UC Davis' Family Practice Residency programs in Sacramento. All of this education took me until 1999, when I finished and returned to Monterey to start in private practice as a Board-Certified Physician in Family Practice.

Upon returning home, I have been involved as Team Physician for Pacific Grove HS, in addition to volunteering for over 15 years in Tournament Headquarters for AT&T Pebble Beach National Pro- AM. Within my scope of Family Medicine, I have trained Resident physicians from the UCSF affiliated Natividad Family Practice Residency Program, trained physicians regarding lipidology and lectured on advanced cardiovascular lab assessment of identifying and treating patients with metabolic syndrome.

I have always believed in a, "healthy mind healthy body" concept as exemplified through my late father who was a tremendous athlete both in swimming and gymnastics while growing up in Romania. His love and passion for water sports rubbed off on our family. While he was a 1st year medical student in Romania, he was threatened by the Communist Party to either join or be killed. He risked his life escaping from Communist Romania in 1948 crossing the frosty shores of the Danube and swimming to freedom in Tito's Yugoslavia. 1 year later he resumed his education in France before eventually coming to the USA on the French quota in the early 1950's. I digressed.

I grew up playing team sports such as baseball, football, and basketball. We had a ping pong table which I spent more time on than anything else. I was introduced to tennis at age 5 but didn't pursue it aggressively until college. Golf is another passion, where I lost myself in the process of attempting to achieve success as well.

A FINAL WORD

Upon three years of preparation, yes, our book was finally finalized for your reading. Having been supposed, imaged, then vaguely visualized in prepublication format during a 30-minute first-lesson for a 4 ½ year old little girl, the literary dream had been realized.

Within minutes of observing talented Kie Foreman, Director of tennis at the Pebble Beach Tennis and Swim Club, neighboring Pacific Grove, Monterey, and Carmel, California, methodically and tenderly guide Juliet Elizabeth of Southern California in the rudimentary steps of a brand-new, special kind of game for her, it enlivened in this co-author several thoughts and questions, all at once: Every child in America, nay, the world, should relish the exhilarating excitement that Juliet was experiencing. Meanwhile, a thousand thoughts raced recklessly along the avenues of my mind assailing all cautious and conservative spending thoughts. All pre-instruction, regardless of cost, should begin, if not the crib or cradle, then certainly by the age of two; that the value of outgoing, expressive, and creative physical recreation for healthy personality growth is incalculable; gentle, gifted, coaching professionals like Kie out there should be the fountainheads of such outdoor learning activities; indeed, Kie should write a book on how he views the lessons of tennis for tots and toddlers, then, those boys and girls between four and give, and from, say, twelve to twenty-one. Yes! Why not, for the first time in the 150-year history of published tennis books, now, worldwide, numbering well over 100,00 write his guide FOR THE PARENTS to direct the action of their own children? And if he's amenable, I'll join him as co-author, having worked with publishers and their editor for more than half a century.

Thus was the birth of our new concept in book publishing.

During the more then 36-40 months that followed, brooding incubation ripening into final vision fruition, we schemed and planned our aims, purposes, the ideas, hopes, and design dreams commingling and coalescing into the first draft of a proposed highly illustrated texted guide for parents. We searched for a sympathetic publisher instead of the usual who relished publishing our effort, if we financed it. We finally agreed upon my own, Creative Texts, which had no such unwarranted, burdensome imposition.

And nearly drowning inundated with recommended book titles and research topics, we focused upon the formatic and fledgling years between 1873, the birth of tennis as we know it, today in Britain, and 1914, the advent of World War I in Europe when all sports ceased to exist. We learned from the tennis-playing authors of those years that because the single most characteristic bearing and behavior of a child, two to four or five, if loved, wanted, and respected, is to learn, anything and everything. Learning is so deeply ingrained in every individual, male or female, that it is almost involuntary, a human species specialized for learning, borne with a "will to learn". If so, wouldn't that include learning the most difficult of all sports, "tennis"? Hence, at two, fun-filled non-stroking games on the court; then, nearing three years, the initial rudiments of pre-skills, the first strokes in the making, grasping, and swinging that feel comfortable in fun and satisfaction activities. And, soon afterwards, the actual hitting strokes.

Thus, because we believe tennis begins in the cradle, our effort to instruct parents how to teach the first never-forgotten lessons of tennis when, "Mommy, daddy, will you teach me to play tennis?" If you believe the first lesson in tennis is "Watch the ball hit the racquet", then surely you will believe, you will echo, the second thought taught by Juan Antonio Chavez Carrillo, a teacher of tennis for more than 30 years and the highly respected Education and Promotion Coordinator for the Mexican Tennis Federation, "If you are a parent, remember that all you have to do to make your child fall in love with tennis for the rest of his life is practice with you. If you are passionate, let him or her play with you and mom. Then, of course, later, as he or she begins to slowly separate from you, place the child with the best certified tennis teaching professional you can find in your area. And, later in life, when asked to play with him or her, always, always agree, smilingly. Then, slowly begin discussion plans of instruction and learning for your grandkids.

And never forget the final lesson of all: Remain passionate about the greatest sport ever conceived.

BIBLIOGRAPHY

Suggested for further reading...incomparable, in a class by itself, highly, highly recommended

A.   Juan Antonio Chavez Carrillo, "Teaching Manual Pre-Tennis, More Than 450 Exercises for Those Who Want to Teach How to Start Playing Tennis or Any Other Racket Sport". Order on Amazon.

B.   Six selected titles from Juan Carrillo's "Teaching Manual Pre-Tennis, More Than 450 Exercises".

- Barrell, M. "Baseline U10. A guide to under 10 junior development"
- Loh, Jim, K I. (1989) "Parent-Player Tennis Training." New York: The Stephen Greene Press.
- USPTA (1986) "The USPTA Junior Development Manual." Westley Chapel, Fl: US Professional Tennis Association.
- USPTA (1998) "The Complete Guide, USPTA Little Tennis." Houston; USPTA.

C.   Thirteen selected titles from Helen Irene Driver's "Tennis For Teachers", 1936.

- Streamline Tennis - Browne, Mary K. - American Sports Publishing Co,

D.   The best tennis books from the 1930s

- "How To Play Tennis" - Mercer Beasley.
- "Budge on Tennis" - Budge, 1939.
- "Tennis, Fundamentals and Timing" - Bruce and Bruce, 1940.
- "Art of Lawn Tennis" - Tilden.
- "Tennis" - Wills
- "Better Tennis" - Wightman.
- "Modern Tennis" - Jacobs.
- "Methods and Players" - Paret.

- "Modern tennis" - Vaile.
- "Psychology and Advanced Play" - Paret.
- "Tennis Tactics" - Little.
- "Match Play and the Spin of the Play" - Tilden.

E.   The Best Tennis Books Between 1873, when tennis was born until the turn of the century

- "100 Years in the Making Australian Open" (1905-2005)
- "Lawn Tennis Supplies" by Horace Partridge
- "Memorandum and Articles of Association of Newcastle district tennis Club Limited"
- "The Fundamentals of Tennis" by Harry Leighton
- "Spalding's Lawn Tennis Guide" (1885)
- "The Modern Method of Training for Running, Walking, Rowing, Boxing, Football, Lawn-Tennis, etc." by Charles Hill

F.   Generally, the best later, and, today, any book with "Tennis" in the title

- Buxton, Angela. Tackle Lawn Tennis This Way. London: Stanley Paul, 1958.
- Harman, Bob. Use Your Head in Tennis. New York: Thomas Crowell, 1974.
- Smyth, John. The Game's the Same - - Lawn Tennis in the World of Sport. New York: Philosophical Library, Inc., 1957.
- Tilden, William T. The Art of Lawn Tennis. Garden City, New York: Garden City Publishing, 1921.
- Walter, Gerald. Your Book of Lawn Tennis. London: Faber and Faber, 1958.
- Seixas, Vic. Prime Tennis: Tennis For Players Over 40. New York: Charles Scribner's Sons, 1983.
- Morton, Jason. Winning Tennis After 40
- Montgomery, Jim. Tennis For the Mature Adult.

"For the child it must be today, now . . . Many other things we need can wait. The little one cannot. Right now is the time his or her bones are being formed, his or her blood is being made, and his senses are being developed. To the child, we cannot answer 'Tomorrow'. His or her name is spelled T O D A Y !"

-Gabriella Mistral, Chilean winner of the Nobel Prize for Poetry

"Education means that the student, even the youngest of the young must be drawn out of the self into other paths . . .This can only be achieved by an educative will . . . No amount of explaining can make the crooked plant grow straight; it must be trained upon the trellis of the norm by the gardener's art . . ."

-Carl Jung

"Always, ever so tenderly, strive toward excellence through critical thinking. Through critical thinking we are achieving excellence, and while we are about it, on the court or at home on the living room floor, we can engage excellence by thinking critically. Back on the court, tennis provides a means to control our game, and, in looking forward, our destiny . . ."

-Kurt Schlesinger, M.D, to his court friends, July 9, 1984, California Tennis Club, San Francisco

In heartfelt remembrance of Maureen Connolly

Her "Hints on Practice and Tournament Play" appeared on page 8 of the 22-page pocket brochure "How to Play Top Notch Tennis, with Official Tennis Rules", published by the Wilson Sporting Goods Co in 1967 and was sold for 35 cents. Other pros offering top tips on how to play championship tennis were Jack Kramer, Tony Trabert, Mary Hardwick and Barry MacKay.

Maureen Connolly

HINTS ON PRACTICE AND TOURNAMENT PLAY

- Practice as much and as often as possible.
- Jump rope to improve your footwork and stamina. Good condition is a prime requisite for a champion.
- Remember to start taking your racket back the instant your opponent hits the ball. Late back swings cause late hitting.
- Try to hit the ball away from your opponent. This will keep him on the defensive.
- If you must move to the far side of the court, get back to the center position quickly.
- Remember to buy good equipment and keep it in first class condition. Personally, I have found Wilson best.
- If you want to improve, watch the better players and enter all tournaments you can.
- Tennis is one of the greatest of international games and is played by more people throughout the world than any other sport.

KEEP YOUR EYE ON THE BALL!

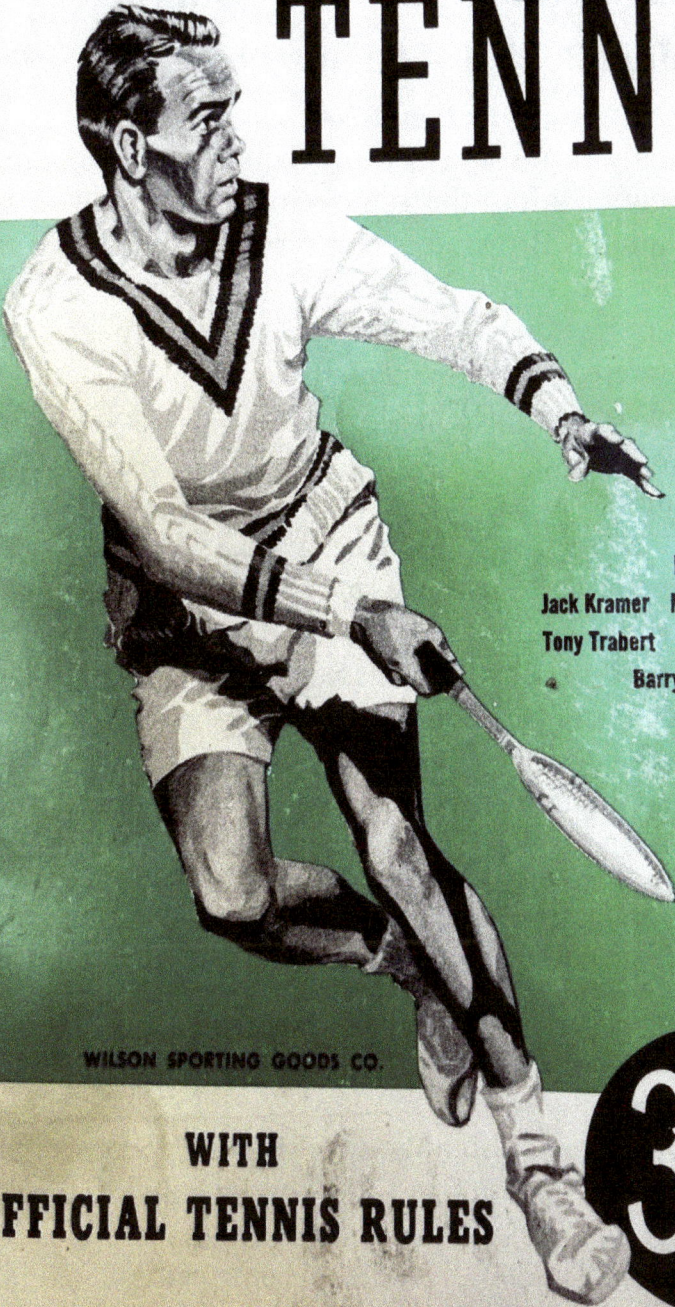

An Expression of Deference, Respect, and Esteem
Mary Kendall "Brownie" Browne
June 3, 1891 – August 19, 1971

-By Don DeNevi

When I accidentally read some of Mary's quotes on tennis for the first time I felt as if a new breath of the game's importance had smacked me, literally. Within a minute Brownie added a new reckoning to my tennis attention, skill, and resoluteness. With additional practice and play, I had to confirm for myself the initial lesson of her Foreword, page 5, in the first of four books she wrote, "Top-Flite Tennis", 1928: "Success lies not so much in genius as in concentrated hard work, plus a love for the game you have chosen to play."

The subtitle, authored by the editors of the American Sports Publishing Company, which Brownie approved, reads, "Practical Instruction Developed from Personal Experience and Taught Successfully by Miss Browne to Her Pupils". Although tiny, 5 ½" x 8 1/8", the 130-page illustrated instructional guide, which, thanks to the Permission Division of the U.S. Copyright Office, in Washington, DC, is presented in its entirety beyond our Appendices- Mary's Gift of Introduction of herself and her teachings to the reader, although 96 years late.

Who was this heroic 5'2" natural athlete winner of 13 major tennis titles, and amateur golfer, this beautiful woman at age 35 in 1926 ranked No. 6 in the world?

Long forgotten, sadly neglected, or simply untaught about or unknown to the much younger tennis generations, allow Brownie in own words on page 5 of her second book, "*Streamline Tennis*", published in 1940, to write of herself-

"My record consists of winning three times the National Singles Champion of the United States; five times the National Ladies' Doubles Champion of our country; nine times National Mixed Doubles Champion in America; Wimbledon Ladies' Doubles Champion in 1926; and twice Captain of the International Wightman Cup team."

From birth, if a smidgen of androgen-producing level of masculine-type play, i.e., fiery-fierce competitiveness, winner take all, death to the loser, existed in some level of her, it never surfaced, ever. Instead, Mary Kendall Browne seemed so fragile, so lovely, so ethereal, everyone, including jealous enemies, wanted to protect her!

That same year, Brownie engaged Suzanne Lenglen, France's supreme tennis prima donna, for a professional tennis tour to 40+ cities across Canada, America, and Cuba. Although friends from the moment they met years before, Mary, having played her six times at Wimbledon, losing all six matches, and Suzanne became best friends, a team envied in the Tennis World. Brownie was crushed, devastatingly, when Suzanne, considered the greatest woman player in the history of tennis at that time, 1938, died suddenly. For decades, when Suzanne Lenglen's name was mentioned, tears welled up in Mary's eyes.

In the 1930s, right up to 7 December 1941, Mary confided to her closest friends she preferred teaching the young girls in America than struggling to win in major championships across Europe, especially when she understood World War II was inevitable. For twelve years, with only one break lasting four years, 1942, 1943, 1944, and 1945, when she reported, first in line, as a volunteer to the home office of the American Red Cross on Monday morning, 8 December 1941, teaching tennis for cities in the public parks, and volunteer work seemed to be her life.

Following her stint as a WWII supervisor of a recovery camp for the American and Allied wounded in Australia, Brownie returned to the United States to teach tennis as a regular instructor at Lake Erie College, Painesville, Ohio, as well as serving as a guest instructor for varying semesters at Stephens College, Missouri; Wilson College, Pennsylvania; Russell Sage College, including high schools, in New York and Maryland, and various other high schools and colleges, public and private for shorter periods. She confided once to close friends that her favorite "college tennis teaching quote" was that found in friend Bill Tilden's latest book, "*Aces, Places, and Faults*". Bill wrote, "In recent years Miss Browne has built up a reputation, well deserved, of being the cleverest and most advanced woman in professional tennis teaching".

But WHO was the real Brownie beneath her cute feminine appearing facial bearing despite always with tennis racquet in hand? Her closest and dearest friends, separately, over decades, answered unabashedly, without reservation or qualification, with essentially the same words: "The sort of unaffected, friendly, always smiling, Touch of Venus, Morning Star, governing her entire being, every day in every way, always typifying the ordinary, easygoing, American happy- go-lucky quiet but spunky young woman you would dearly want to bring home to meet mom, dad, and family".

Her instinct was to teach tennis to anyone, male and female, alone or in groups, of any age who would listen, eager to learn, knowing instinctively the game would add years to one's life, and his or her happiness. If the uninterested turned their backs, she again smiled, never confusing independence of thought with discourteousness. While a zest for life was always apparent in her effervescence, not to be confused with vivaciousness, so was a deeply hidden sadness she only confided to her closest friends, Suzanne being one, "I'm afraid I was designed for spinsterhood".

To this moment, for me, what stands out the most was her quiet fortitude, resilience, and brilliance of writing, every sentence echoing the feeling that life is somehow incomplete without tennis. Like sunshine every morning.

Read her writings for yourself. It's your gift, either one to cherish, or one to pass on to the avid, or soon to be.

A Surprise Gift

from

Mary K.

Browne

3 Times National Singles

5 Times National Ladies Doubles Champion

and

Twice Captain of the International Wightman Cup Team

MARY K. BROWNE

TOP-FLITE TENNIS

by

Mary K. Browne

Former

National Women's Singles Champion

National Women's Doubles

Champion

Captain Wightman Cup Team

Practical instruction developed from personal experience and taught successfully by Miss Browne to her pupils

__DEDICATION__

I dedicate this book to the *Game of Tennis.* So finely conceived that
"time cannot change nor custom stale its infinite variety."
-Mary K. Browne

*Success lies not so much in genius as in concentrated hard work,
plus a love for the thing you are doing.*

ATHLETIC SPORT AS A TRAINING SCHOOL FOR LIFE

I believe there is no better way to train youngsters in the art of facing and defeating the problems of life than through the medium of athletic sports.

If they have acquired any degree of success at their game, they have learned all the essential qualities of sportsmanship and discipline which will contribute substantially to their success in business.

The story of so many successful businessmen is the story of many successful athletes:

An aptitude rather than any startling genius.

A capacity for work.

A love for the thing that they are doing.

A focus of thought an energy.

A "desire to win only outweighed by a determination to play fair."

INTRODUCTION

In this book on tennis instruction, I hope to make a simple explanation of the game, so that it will give to the average tennis enthusiast a clear understanding of the first principles of tennis.

The most important task before me is to help you *visualize* the game of tennis. To see in your mind's eye what you are striving for. You need not know all the results of certain actions so long as you visualize and execute that action accurately. Probably only one in every thousand persons who drive an automobile knows the intricacies of its machinery. They know how to start, guide, and stop it; for all practical purposes, they need know no more.

So, in the tennis stroke, if you know how to start, guide, and stop your stroke you need not necessarily know all the surrounding and sustaining phenomena. The strokes directed in a certain specific manner get the results for certain complicated reasons. It is the simple direction and not the complicated reasons to which I wish most to direct your attention. Then you will initiate the action which will get the results.

I have departed from the usual photographic illustrations of good form for the line drawings *(which were taken from actual photographs)*. These drawings show more clearly the specific points to be explained, because just as every motion behind the footlights must be exaggerated to attract and hold attention, I have had these points emphasized in the line drawings.

I have purposely left out of this book the "chop" stroke because it has proved itself an unworthy stroke as the basis of good tennis form. Since it is conceded only the position as an ornament to the game and because of the amount of energy expended in acquiring this stroke and the risk involved in using it, there seems very little use to consider it in the first stages of a tennis career.

Suzanne Lenglen, the greatest woman tennis player in the world, scarcely ever uses the chop; nor does Helen Wills, our present national champion. Mrs. Mallory, who has been champion of the United States seven times, literally never uses it. In the games of the best men the chop plays a very small role. Ninety-five per cent of the ground strokes are drives.

It seems that in most athletic pursuits, certainly in swimming, riding and golf, and on the dance floor, children are schooled in what is the correct form. They take pride in knowing how to handle the double reins of the English bridle and to rise gracefully and rhythmically to the trot. They are not satisfied to be able to keep on top of the water in the swimming tank, they must stroke in good form. Yet upon the tennis court they are allowed to go at the game any old way, pushing, shoving, scarcely ever stroking or timing the tennis ball.

The actual tennis stroke is very easy to acquire. Simplicity is the essence of its good form. It is much easier to connect with the tennis ball and to cope with the vast variety of bounds with the drive stroke, but it does not seem to be natural for beginners to go at the game with the side stroke or the drive. In fact, I am of the opinion that correct form in games is not the natural way. The overlapping grip in golf, for example. The correct tennis grips will feel awkward at first, but the muscles will soon fall in line and there will be no strain whatsoever.

GRIPS

It is absolutely essential in the proper production of the strike to assume the correct grip for each of the various strokes.

There are three distinct grips. One for the forearm, one for the backhand, and one for the service.

Since there is a different grip for each one of these strokes, it involves a definite shift of the hand on the racket handle.

The three positions of the hand on the racket shown in the drawings on following page are the grips used by the best players today.

They are fundamentally correct.

Slight individual variation is permissible but to stray far will produce a freak grip and freakish results.

The octagonal shape of the handle helps *feel* for the grip when shifting and serves also in keeping the hand from slipping.

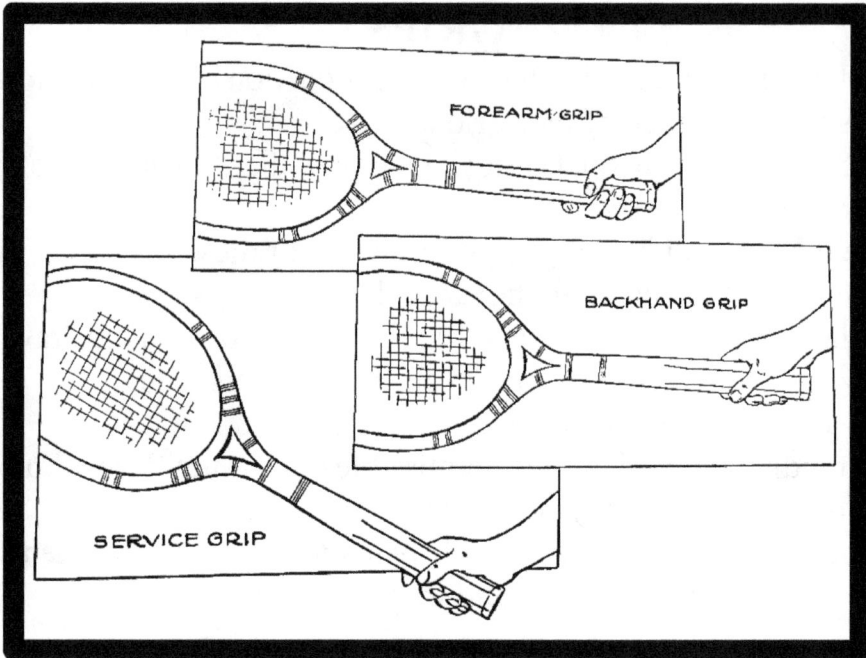

Forearm Grip
Note position of thumb in relation to octagonal-shaped handle.

Backhand Grip
Follow position of thumb. Note that it is further around the handle, bringing the hand more on top of the handle. (This grip used also for the Backhand Volley.)

Service Grip
Note position of thumb on handle. This grip is just between the forearm and the backhand grips. (This grip used also for the Forearm Volley and Overhead Smash.)

TILT OF THE RACKET FACE

In order to accomplish a clean hit ball, you must have some conception of what a variety of results you can obtain by the simple tilt of the face of your racket.

It is essential to understand its effect upon your shot.

In golf, you have sometimes as many as fifteen clubs, the main difference, one form the other, being in the loft on the face of the club, which gives various flights and spins to your ball.

In *Tennis*, you have *one* racket, which must serve for all types of shots.

The *Flat* face contacts the ball straight and sends it off on more or less of a straight line.

The *Open* face is tiled back in order to loft the ball in the air.

The *Closed* face is turned toward the ground and is used only at the finish of a stroke to bring a ball down from a height.

THE SHIFT

The *Shift*, which is changing the position of the hand on the racket when going from the forearm to the backhand stroke or vice versa, must *always* be accomplished before meeting the ball. Sometimes it must be accomplished in a hurry.

The skillful players of today have improved the manner of shifting, which leaves no doubt as to its great advantage over the old way.

In the *new* way of *shifting*, you bring your racket *straight* across in front of the body, shifting the hand on the racket handle.

The *opposite* face of your racket meets the ball.

The *old* way the racket was brought *up* across the body, *turned* over and the *same* face of the racket met the ball.

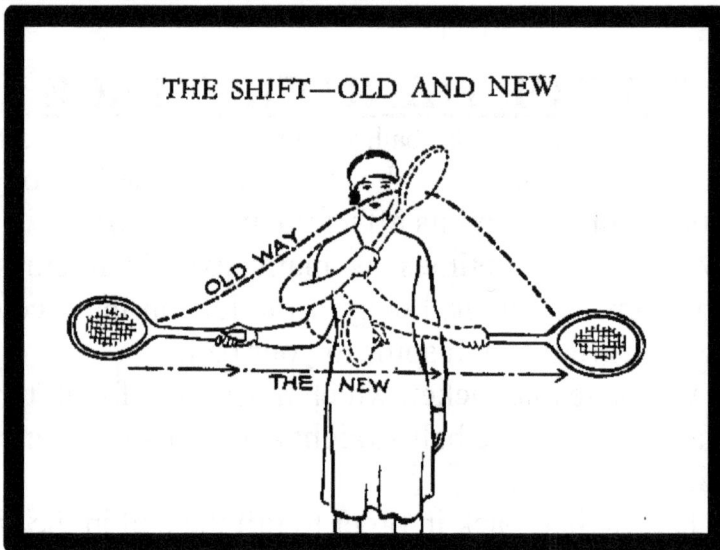

THE SHIFT—OLD AND NEW

You will note in the drawing illustrating the new and old shift that the new way brings the racket into position in a straight line, which has always been the shortest distance between two points, therefore the fastest shift and for that reason the best.

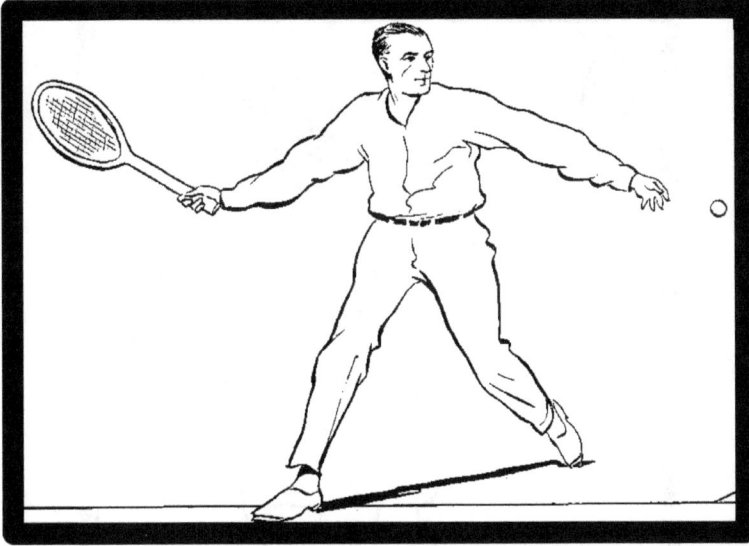

WILLIAM M. TILDEN...... Preparedness at its best.
Perfect example of getting the racket back long before the arrival of the ball.

PREPAREDNESS

Preparedness contributes more to the success of your stroke than any one other thing, *because* if you start right, you can finish right.

Being prepared seems to contribute to correct balance, proper timing and a good finish.

My theory—which is no longer a theory, but a practical success among my pupils—is that you should *prepare* for your strike well in advance of the arrival of the ball, so that you can make a long strike, which is necessary in returning the ball form one end of the court to the other without being hurried.

If you wait until the last moment to get your racket back, you are hurried and at the most can flick an ineffective racket at the ball.

You can maneuver into position just as well with your racket back as with it forward.

As soon as you know whether your return will be a backhand or a forearm stroke, then your racket should go immediately in the back position.

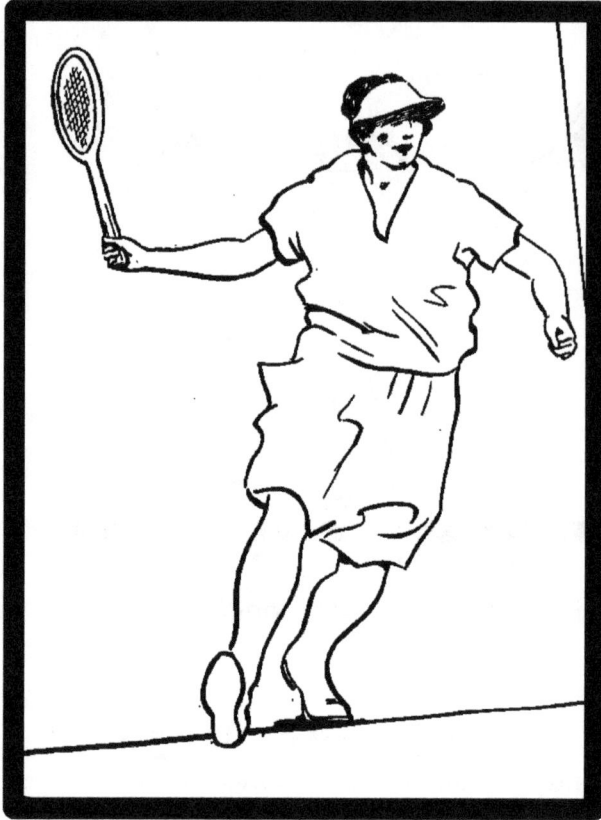

HELEN WILLS.......Prepared

Her racket back while she is still running into position to drive the ball

Get to your back position in the quickest, least complicated way without flourishes.

The illusion has existed for years that a tennis drive stroke is all one continuous motion.

IT IS NOT!

The backswing should be entirely detached from the forward stroke, giving you the opportunity to concentrate on getting into position and being the personification of deliberation in making your stroke.

It is indefinitely easier to time the ball correctly if you take your racket back to a stationary position and hit from there.

If you wait with your backswing, in an effort to make your drive stroke all one continuous motion, you are obliged to sense the exact moment to start your backswing in order to connect exactly with the forward swing and then not meet your ball too soon nor too late. It complicates an otherwise simple stroke.

Since there is *no* reason why we should make a DRIVE stroke all one continuous motion, you cannot but agree that it is easier and better in every way to separate your backswing from your forward swing.

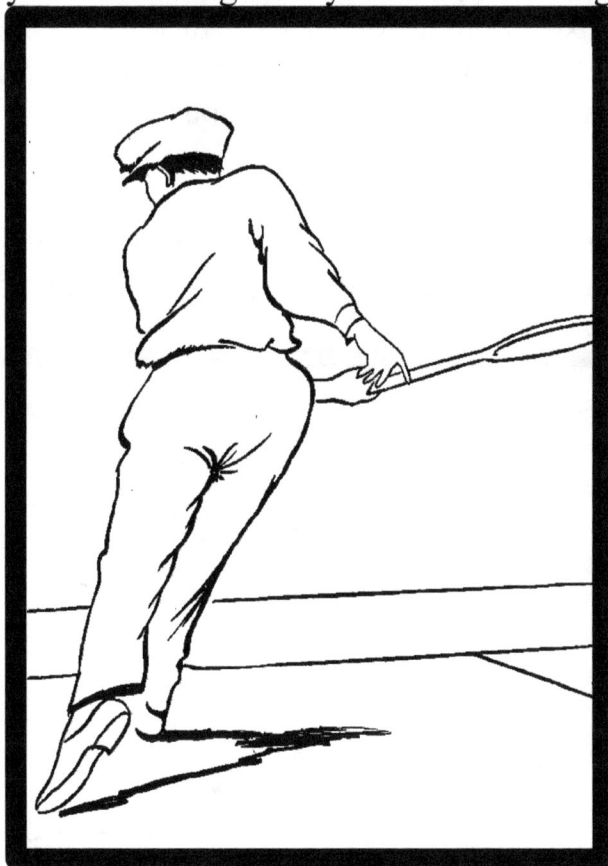

NORMAN E. BROOKES……. Prepared
Racket back long before the arrival of the ball.

The Exception

The only criticism I have ever heard advanced against this method, with Preparedness as its foundation, and the immediate and detached backswing as the vital part of Preparedness, is that on a very short ball just over the net, you cannot reach it if you run with your racket back.

As there are exceptions to every rule, to retrieve the short, close-in returns you run with your racket extended in FRONT of you. This increases your reach, and on these occasions only a very short poke is necessary to return the ball the shorter distance over the net into your opponent's court.

I have found no trouble with my pupils in their ability to handle the combination of deep and short balls, getting the racket back, or forward, as the stroke demands.

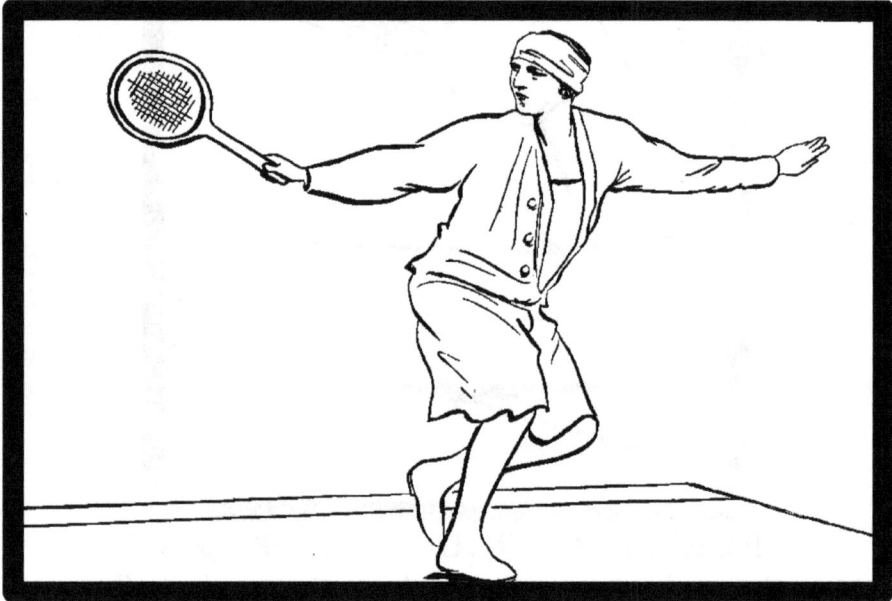

SUANNE LENGLEN....... Fine finish to the backhand drive.
Suzanne finishes high and with that face of the racket. She uses the "thumb up the handle" grip. Note beautiful balance.

THE ELABORATE FLOURISH vs. THE SIMPLE, DIRECT ROUTE

The inclination of most tennis players is to be elaborate in taking their rackets back. They describe beautiful arcs, sometimes going forward and then back, turning their rackets over and twirling them in their hands.

These unnecessary motions may all be in the great cause of lines and curves, but it too often results in stroking the tennis ball with artistic hands and wrists rather than the more effective athletic muscles.

If you are elaborate in your backswing and roll your wrist, then you must unwind the elaborateness by the time you are ready to stroke the ball, so that the flat or straight face of your racket will meet the ball. You complicate an otherwise simple motion.

The better way is the simple and direct route.

Fling your racket back without flourishes and with some force, so that you will get to the back position quickly and correctly. Make it a habit on all long returns.

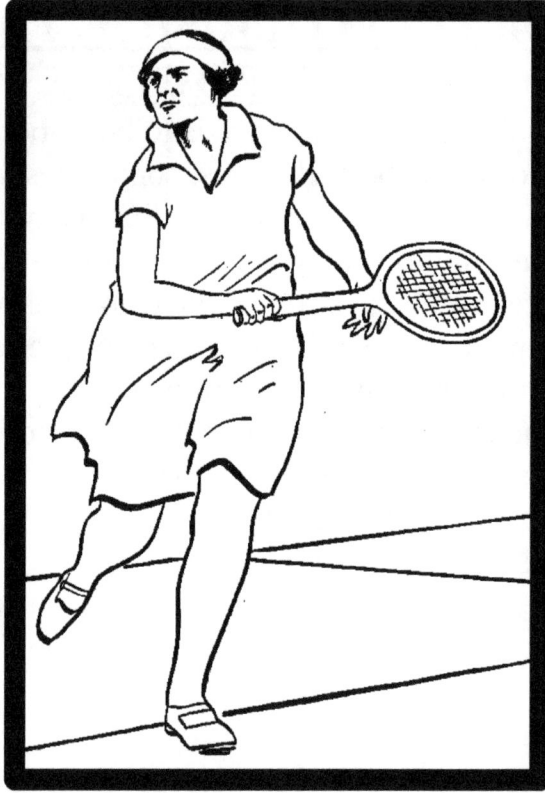

BETTY NUTHALL....... Preparedness exaggerated

Very conspicuous in her ground strokes; the distinct separation of back swing from forward swing.

PREPARATION FOR THE FULL DRIVE STROKE

As soon as the mind registers whether the stroke will be played from the forearm or backhand—

Assume the correct grip—

Take your racket back *at once* to the limit of the backswing, long before arrival of the ball, and hold it there stationary. The face of the racket *flat*.

Maneuver into position—

Turn the body sideways to the net—

Get your weight back at the beginning of the stroke.

Simplicity is always good form and good taste. It is that, and more, in tennis. It is good judgment as well, for often it saves the fraction of a second, which makes the difference between a good stroke and a poor, hurried one.

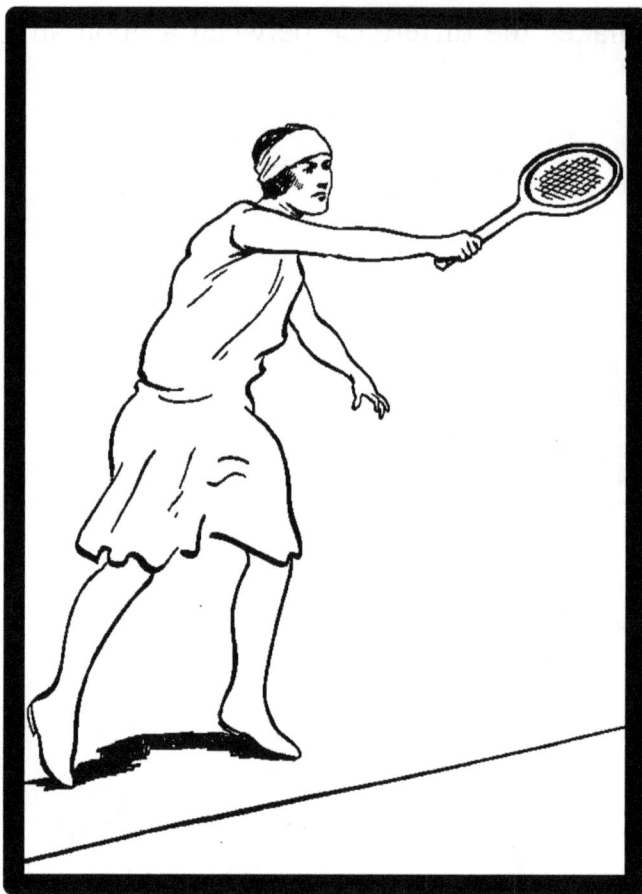

SENORITA LILA d'ALVARE.....A fine finish to a forearm drive.

EXECUTING THE FOREARM DRIVE STROKE

As you start your *forward* swing, grip your racket firmly.

Look at the ball until you hit it.

Get into position so that you can meet the ball at your side.

The average drive should be struck when the ball is about waist high.

Follow through as far as possible in line with the intended flight of the ball.

Let the racket turn over easily at the end of the swing.

Finish with a long follow-through.

Let your weight come forward as though you intended to go on into the net.

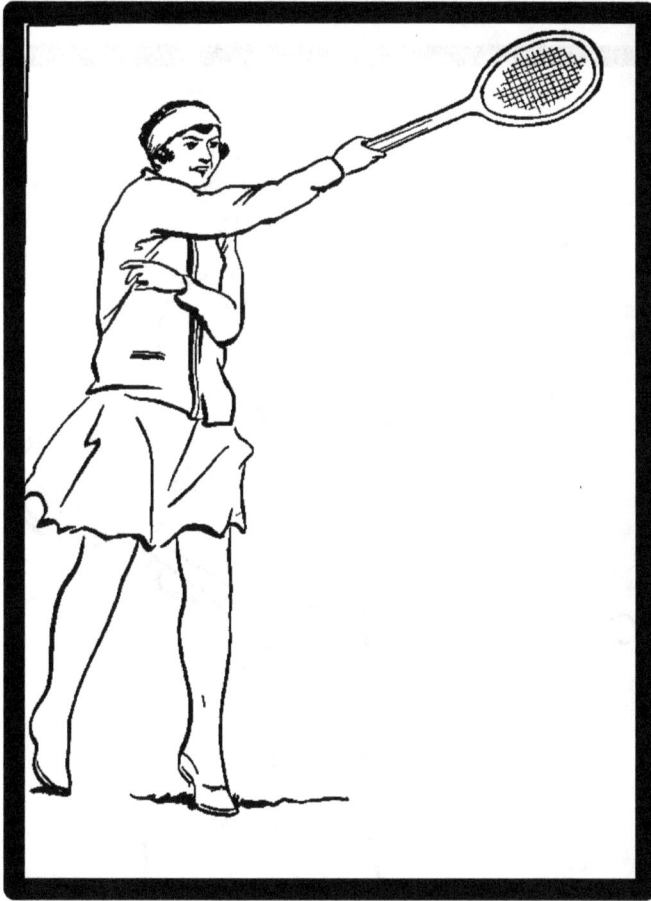

BETTY NUTHALL'S….. *Finish to her forearm drive*
The long follow-through gives her return fine depth and pace off the surface of the court.

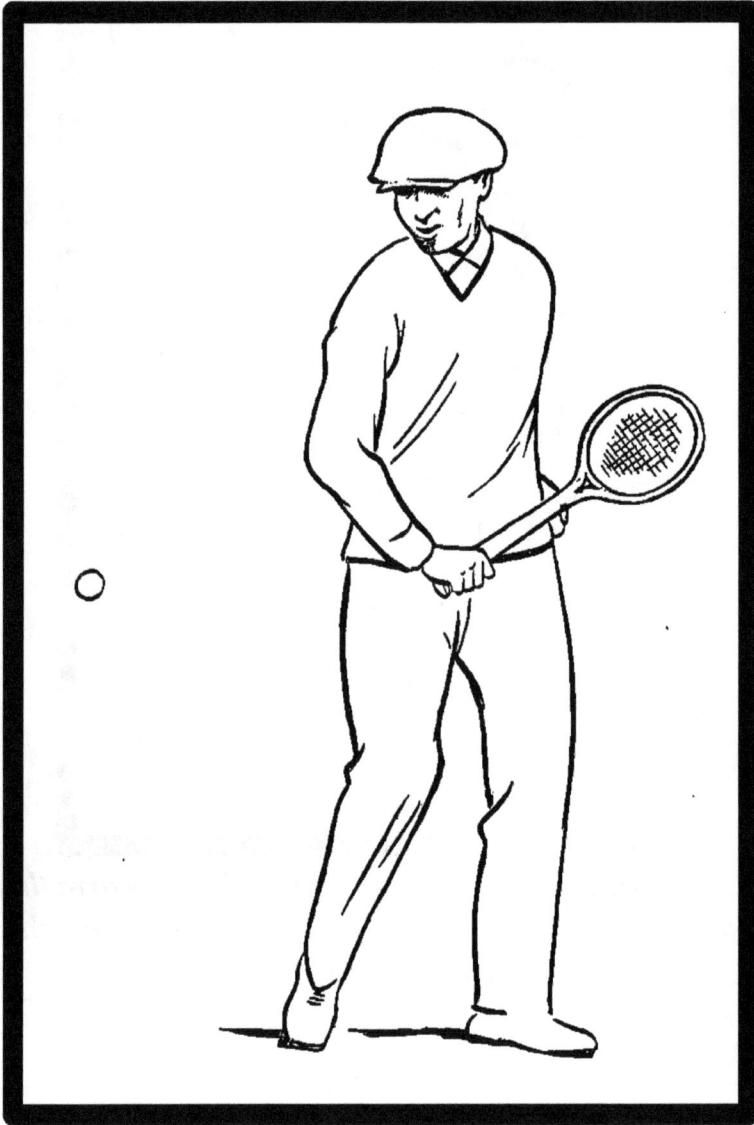

RENE LACOSTE……. Fine example of Preparedness
Racket back long before the arrival of the ball; weight back, and he has turned sideways to make his stroke.

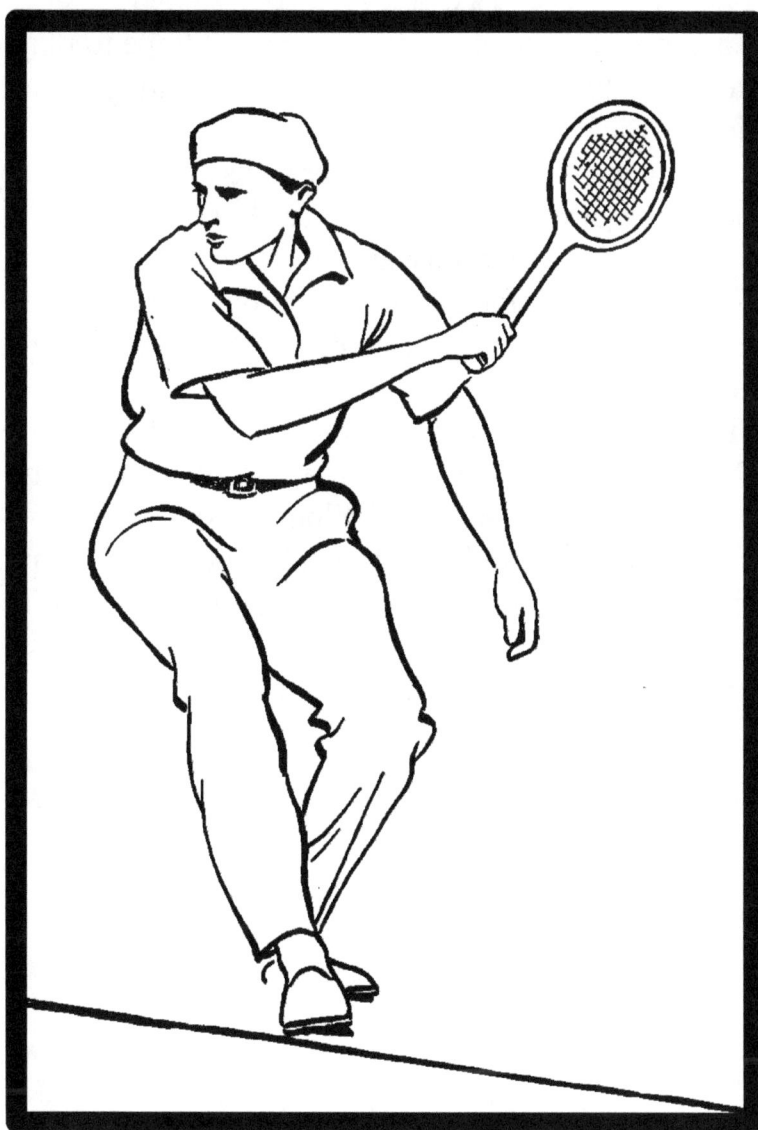

JEAN BOROTRA.....Prepared

While still moving into position. You can be too late, but never too soon, with your backswing.

ACTIVITY

Tennis is a game of great activity. You cannot hope to play unless you are willing and capable of moving quickly and with judgment into the correct relation to your ball.

It is best to cultivate the shorter, quicker steps of the boxer, to keep your feet close enough together when you are ready to stroke, so that you can get your weight back, and then forward, into the stroke.

If your feet are spread far apart your body weight is heavily in the center. You cannot get it back, or forward, into the stroke. You can scarcely get it up to continue the play.

William Tilden learned to skip just as he reached striking position, so as to bring his feel closer together at the end of a long run, when it is sometimes necessary to leap and to take long strides to cover the distance.

Don't leave your feet behind and stretch for the ball if it is possible with a quicker start and faster moving to get to the ball well poised for your stroke.

Skipping rope is good training for footwork.

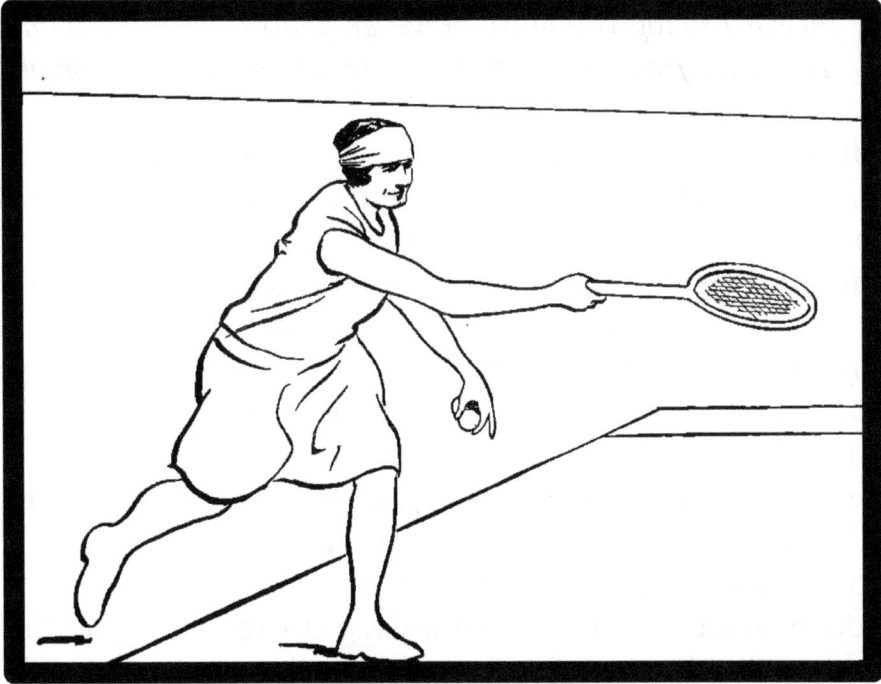

LILA d'ALVAREZ…..Beautiful finish for the low-bounding back-court drive

Finish with the open face to give loft to the ball in order to help clear the net.

MOMENTUM AND THE FINISH

The drive in tennis is unlike the golf swing in that in tennis you are going forward to meet a *lively* ball which has speed and needs only to be returned at the very most not over thirty yards. All that is necessary to send back the ball at terrific speed that distance is the forward swing.

In golf you are playing a *lifeless* ball and momentum of the club head must be worked up by one continuous swing in order to send the ball the hundreds of yards required in a golf game.

The service stroke in tennis is the only stroke where a lifeless ball is struck, and in that stroke, as in the golf swing, it should be continuous, and the momentum developed by describing a large continuous arc.

In the forward swing you must, however, follow through, in either golf or tennis. The finish means everything. It gives control, direction and depth to the tennis stroke.

The finish is gauged by whether you are trying to bring down a high bound or lift the low bound over the net, also the direction you wish your return to take.

On the high bound, with the ball hit when it is higher than the net, your racket at the backswing is higher than the waist but lower than the ball and is brought up over the ball with the finish across the body and down. The face of the racket is "closed"; that is, it is turned over and the face of the racket which contacted the ball is pointed toward the ground.

In the low bound the backswing is kept lower than the bound and the finish is higher and out from the body. The face of the racket which hit the ball is "open" and more or less facing the sky.

The drive stroke in tennis is not a wrist stroke where you flick your racket at the ball. Move the flat face of the racket on the ball with a firm wrist, moving forearm, shoulder and body all together, thus bringing into the stroke the big muscles and body weight.

LOOK AT THE BALL UNTIL YOU HIT IT!

Clean hitting—in fact, connecting with the ball at all—means that you must

LOOK
AT THE
BALL
UNTIL
YOU
HIT
IT!

The peculiar connection between the vision and the accurate co-ordination of the muscles perhaps you will appreciate if you try to drive a nail without looking at the nail until you hit it.

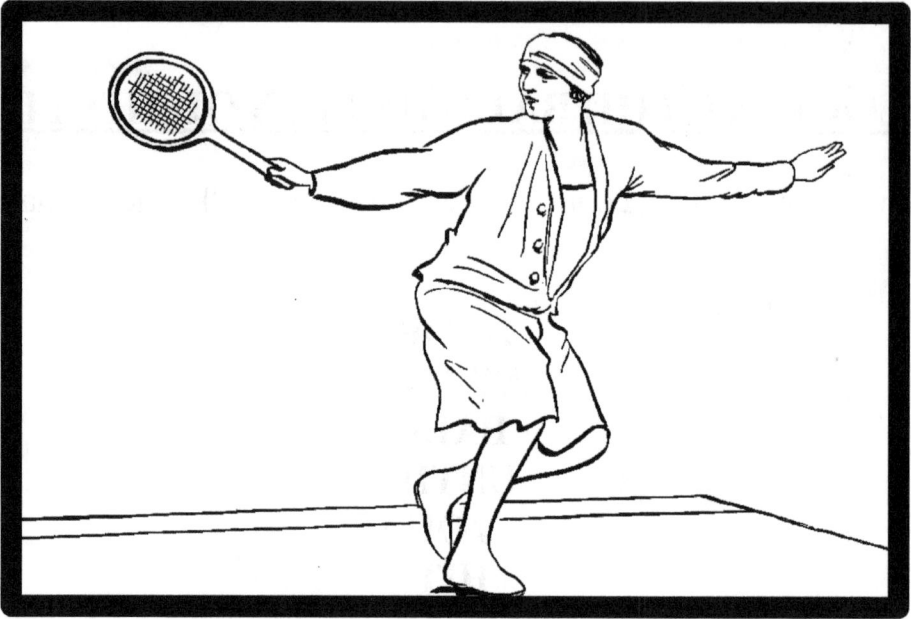

SUZANNE LENGLEN....... Fine finish to the backhand drive.
Suzanne finishes high and with that flat face of the racket. She uses the "thumb up the handle" grip. Note beautiful balance.

THE BACKHAND DRIVE STROKE

The preparation for the backhand drive is practically the same as for the forearm.

Take your racket back long before arrival of the ball.

Keep the face of the racket flat and head of your racket up above the wrist.

Maneuver into position, turning sideways to the net.

Detach backswing from forward swing.

Start your stroke lower than the bound.

Let the ball come down waist high.

Finish high.

Follow through in the direction you wish the ball to take.

Do not turn your racket over as you do in the forearm finish but keep the face of your racket flat.

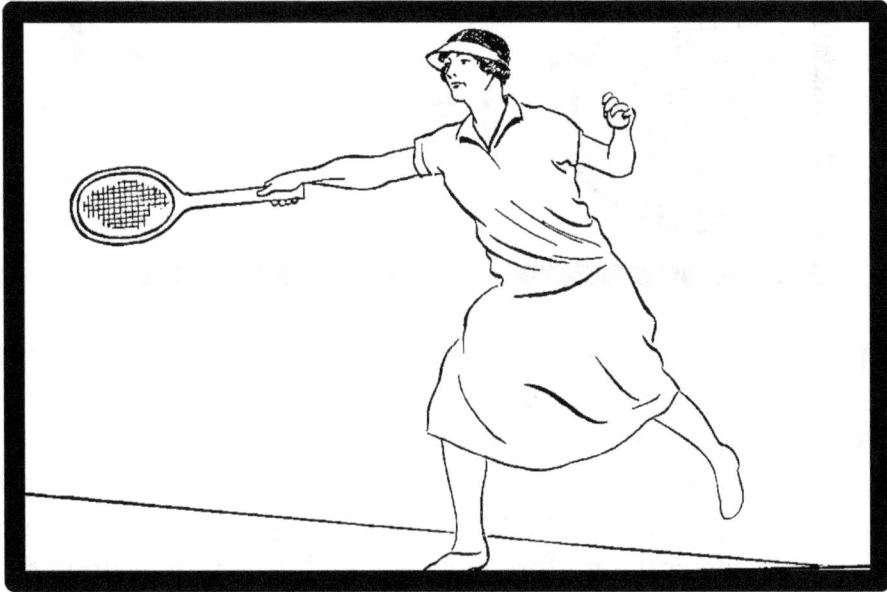

HELEN WILLS'.....Finish to full backhand stroke

Helen uses the 'thumb up the handle' grip. Note that the racket has not been turned over at the finish. The long "follow through" out from the body gives depth and pace to her stroke.

BACKHAND GRIP, WITH THUMB UP THE HANDLE

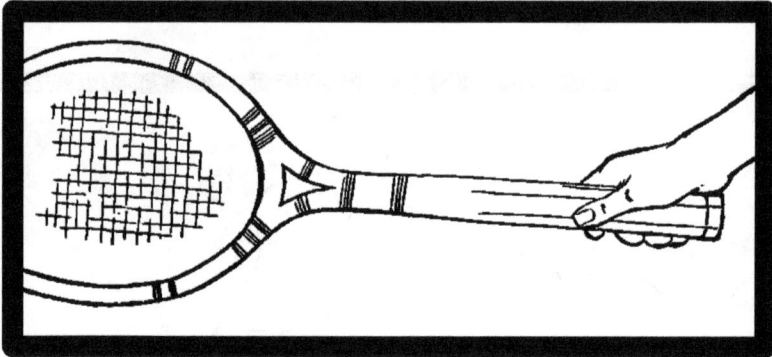

The position of the hand is exactly the same on the handle as the regular backhand grip. The thumb is put up the handle instead of around.

There is no reason why you cannot stroke as freely, easily and accurately from the backhand as from the forearm, if you will turn sideways so that you get the body out of the way. You bring your racket arm on the left side and therefore have as much freedom as upon the right wing.

If you are careful to shift your grip, you will have as much power in your stroke.

Many first-class players are steadier, if not as severe, from their backhand as from the forearm.

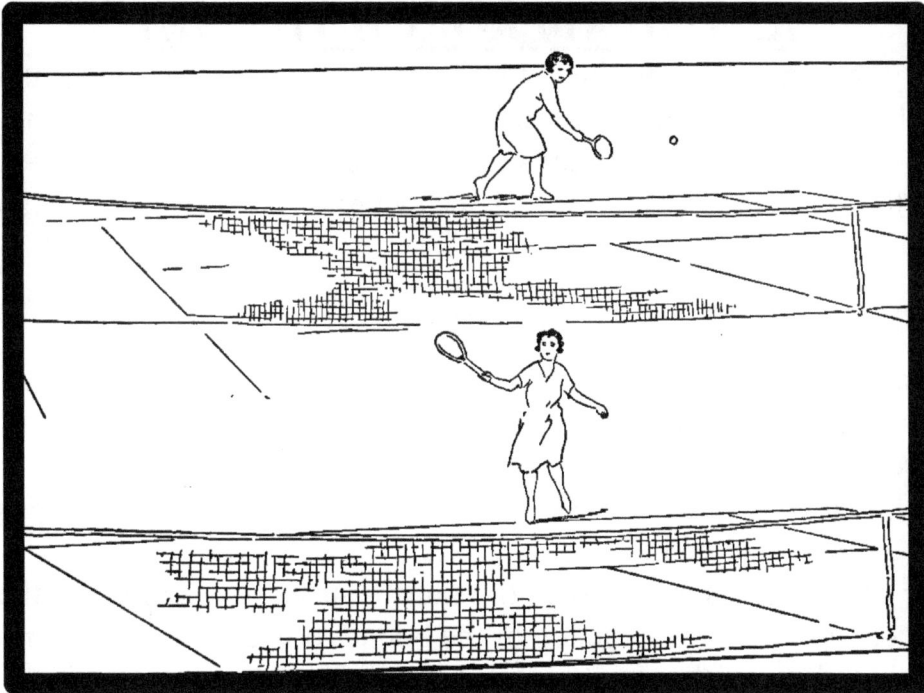

LIFTING THE LOW BALL

The drawings (above) were made to illustrate the LOW backswing and HIGH finish.

This is to ensure a low ball to rise over the net. Note that the flat face of the racket is presented to the ball and the face which contacts the ball is not turned toward the ground, as in the finish for the forearm, but is perpendicular to the ground at the finish of this backhand stroke.

It is essential to let the ball come down from the top of the bound on the backhand and to keep your backswing LOW and finish HIGH.

AS YOU APPROACH THE NET

As you come closer to the net a shortened swing is required, just as in golf when one approaches the green. The swing is shortened, and the body is turned less sideways. When we come practically on top of the net to return the swift volley, there is *no* backswing; the stroke is all forward.

TIMING

Timing, we have always been told, is important in any athletic feat. It is of the greatest importance in the tennis stroke. Which is timing and how do we do it?

To begin with, almost everyone hurries his stroke. Hurry into position but be deliberate in making your stroke.

For *all* beginners it is best to time one's stroke so as to strike the ball after it comes down form the top of the bound. It is especially important to let the ball down if the stroke is taken on the backhand, for one has little power in stroking shoulder high on the backhand.

A ball can be returned, even though it is within a few inches of the ground; therefore, if you find yourself too near or too far away from the ball when you would ordinarily want to stroke it, sidestep it or step nearer, as the requirement may be, taking the extra time to move into position. You will make a better stroke than if you tried to strike the ball at the first possible moment, regardless of your position.

You have much more time than you think to stroke the majority of returns. Take your time. The exact moment to strike is one which is individual. It is something the player must sense, just as one would to keep in time with music.

When you send off a clean hit and speedy ball with very little effort, then you have timed your ball properly; for it is timing more than brute force, which secures speed.

While the timing of the tennis stroke is so individual that no two players time the ball exactly alike, still there are three accepted times when the tennis ball may be stroked with good results. Each, however, has its particularly good points, its disadvantages and its risks.

The three recognized times to stroke the ball are

—On the *rise*.

—On the top of the *bound*.

—On the *descent.*

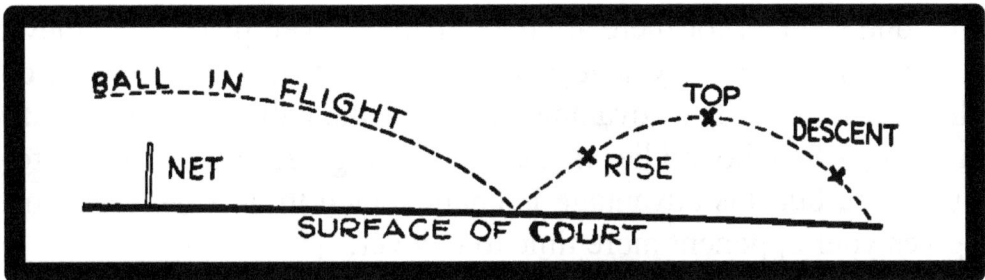

On the rise

The ultra-modern way and only safe in the hands of the most skilled, because you must be exceedingly fleet of foot, keen of eye and possessed of rare judgment. The ball retains all its speed and spin, and you give yourself less time to get into position, making the risk great.

The advantage is in that you can return the ball sooner to your opponent's court, giving him less time to recover; also you need use less of your strength in making a fast return and thus save your energy. You can play closer in the court and therefore cover your court more readily. The clever, alert and agile Frenchmen take the ball on the rise, whenever possible.

On Top of the Bound

This is the timing made famous by the Californians. It is less risky than taking the ball on the rise, but it requires speed of foot to get to your ball in time to take it on top. The advantage lies in that you return the ball sooner to your opponent's court than if you allowed it to come down below the top, and you usually stroke the ball while it is higher than the net and can, therefore, bring it down into your opponent's court with greater force.

On the Descent

The timing which is easiest to learn, and which is absolutely essential to everyone's game, for there are many balls so well placed that they can only be reached when they have come very close to the surface of the court for the second time. The advantage in taking the ball after it comes down from the top of the bound lies in the fact that it gives you more time to get into position, but this advantage is counteracted to an extent, because it also gives your opponent more time to recover.

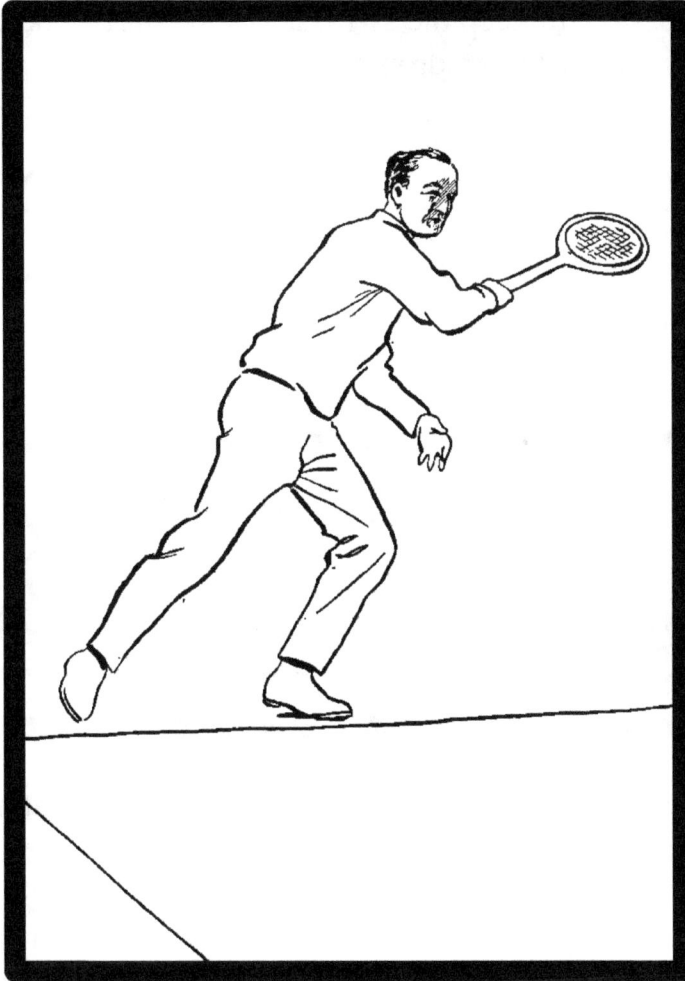

WILLIAM JOHNSTON….. at the end of his famous *'Top-Spin'* drive

TOP OR FORWARD SPIN ON THE FLAT DRIVE

There exists a delusion among some good tennis players that the *flat* drive does not carry top spin. It does.

The ball is contacted with the straight or flat face of the racket, but the *up*-and-*over* plane of the stroke causes the ball to spin forward, and it therefore has top spin.

There are simply different degrees of spin, and the flat drive is a species of drive which carries very little spin. It carries some, though, for it would be almost impossible to keep the swift drives in court if they did not have the forward spin to give them drop.

THE TOP-SPIN vs. THE CHOP

The top-spin drive is better adapted to the tennis game than the chop or undercut drive.

The top-spin drive describes a graceful and *safe* arc when clearing the net, affording less risk of making an error by netting the ball,

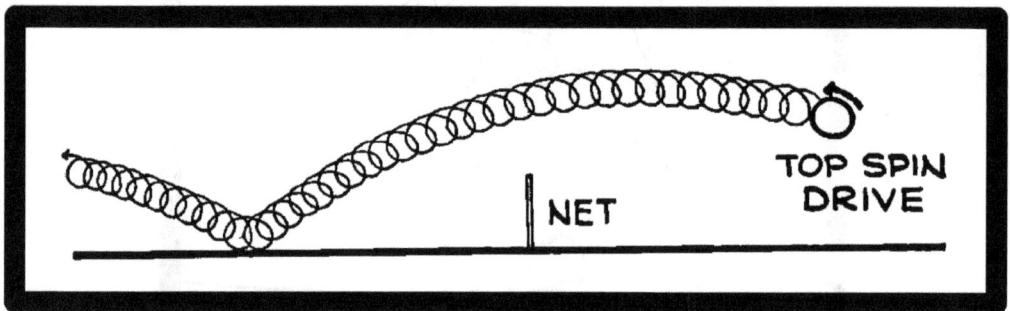

while the chop or undercut drive sails in more or less of a straight line and must be played close to the top of the net to keep the stroke in bounds, for the cut ball drops only when its speed is spent. The over-spin of the top drive will cause a ball to drop, even though it is hit with terrific force.

Besides the fact that the top-spin drive is safer than the chop, it also is far more difficult to handle after it strikes the surface of the court because it carries far greater pace. The chop or undercut drive comes off the surface of the court with its speed checked by the back-spin, which makes it infinitely easier to stroke as soon as one discovers which way it is apt to shy. This can be very easily handled by getting close to where the ball bounds so that you can reach it readily, for, regardless of which way it is

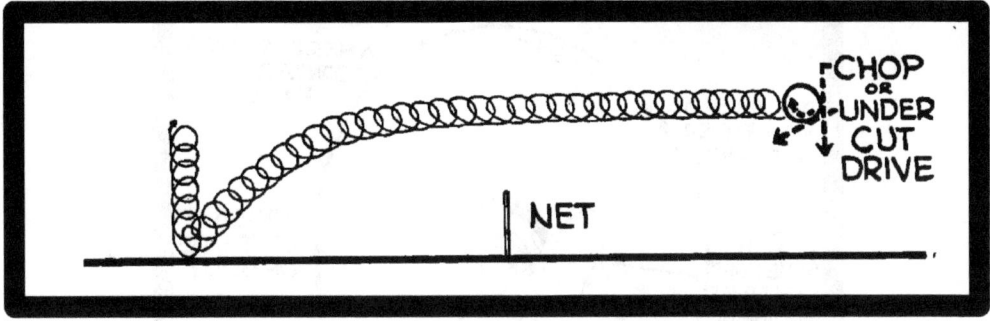

CHOP OR UNDER CUT DRIVE

NET

cut, it will hang for you in the air, while the top-spin drive will shoot so rapidly from the surface of the court that it is far more difficult to handle.

The two shots act very much like the topped mashie to the green in golf, which will shoot off the green because of its over-spin, while the back-spin mashie, which corresponds to the chop, will bite the green and stop.

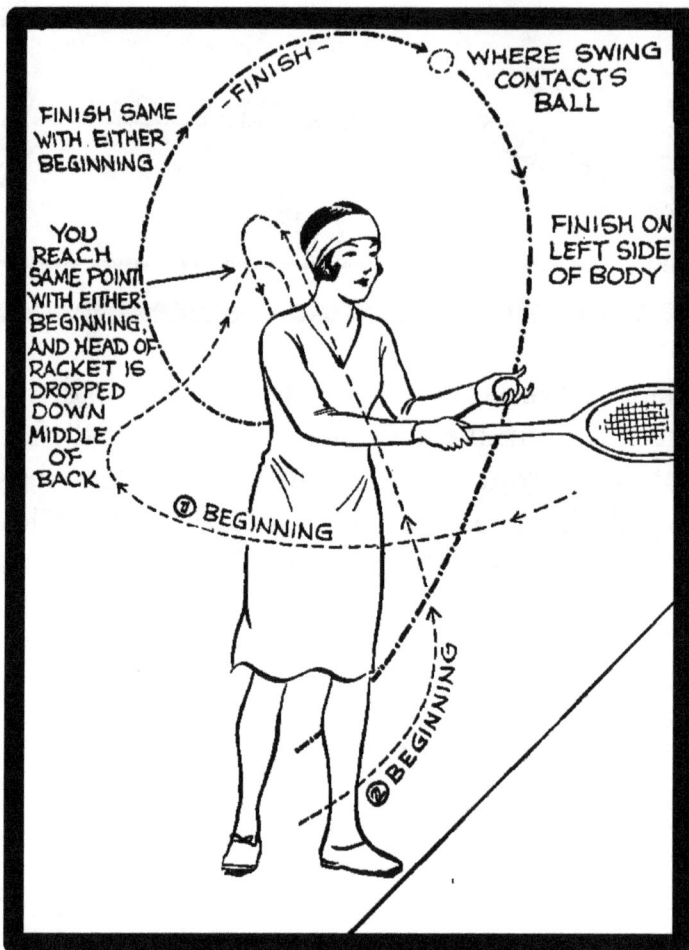

This service swing is like swinging Indian clubs. The grip must be relaxed, the wrist broken and arm bent so the head of the racket can drop down middle of back. The grip is tightened on forward swing.

THE SERVICE

There are various types of services, but I shall describe the one most universally used.

Beginning No. 1 is most graceful.

Beginning No. 2 is easiest for beginners to get their timing.

You can reach point where racket is dropped down the back with either beginning and it does not matter which you choose, but you *must* finish correctly and *there is only one finish.*

At the beginning of the service the body should be turned sideways, with the left shoulder pointing toward your opponent's service court.

It is important now to get your right foot too far behind your left, as you would then lose your balance on your forward swing.

The service grip brings the end of the racket pointing toward the service court, with the face of the racket perpendicular to the ground.

SUZANNE LENGLEN....With racket dropped down her back,
just beginning the finish of her service. Note that she is up on her toes in order to strike the ball at the limit of her extended reach. The position of her feet is correct for easy balance.

The tendency with the first few stroked played with this grip is to careen sharply to the left until you have become accustomed to directing the racket on the ball at the top of the stroke.

The weight is back at the beginning of the service and forward at the finish.

In this particular service the ball should be thrown toward the right shoulder and slightly in front of the body. It should be thrown slightly in advance of the swing of the racket and sufficiently high to give the racket time to gather speed.

The racket is taken up and the head of the racket dropped down the back and then swung forward in an effort to hit the ball at the very top of the reach and toward the top end of the face of the racket.

The finish should be down and across the left side of the body.

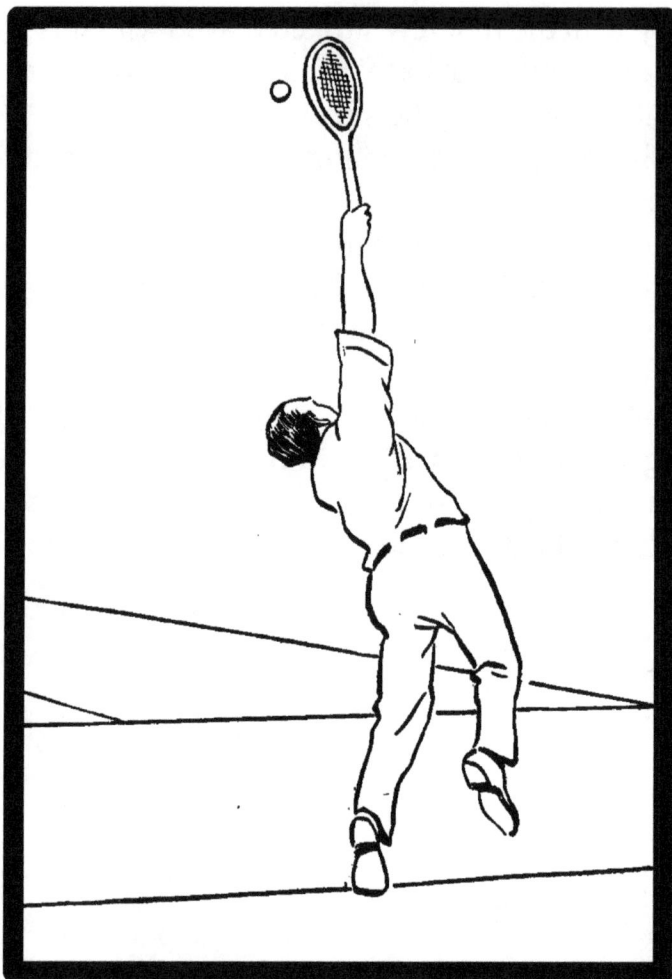

MAURICE McLOUGHLIN…..At the top of his powerful service.

TOSSING THE BALL FOR SERVICE

Tossing the ball consistently well is difficult even for many of the experts. It requires a good deal of concentration. The toss should be made mainly with the wrist; the arm moves only slightly upward. If you let your arm wander up it will toss the ball back of the head and if you let the ball leave your fingers too soon it will fly too far forward; therefore, you must bring into play the same snap of the wrist and release of the ball as the baseball pitcher handles his wrist and fingers. Practice tossing the ball into the air, first rather low, then higher and higher, *without* bringing up the arm only slightly. You will soon acquire accuracy, which is third per cent of a good service.

In the McLoughlin illustration on opposite page note the extended reach and his position on his toes—striking the ball at the highest possible position, which makes it easier to clear the net and keep the service in bounds. Also note way face of racket has changed, from being *perpendicular to ground* at beginning to *facing ground* as it comes on to the ball. Height of stature is a very distinct advantage of service.

A twist is given the ball, which keeps it in bounds. There is a great advantage in being tall because it is easier to bring a ball down from a height, clear the net and keep it in bounds than if it goes off at a lower trajectory. The twist given the ball starts it first on an upward flight and then it takes a sudden drop, which greatly helps in avoiding the net and still keeping it in the bounds of the service court. William Johnson has the best service of any short player I know.

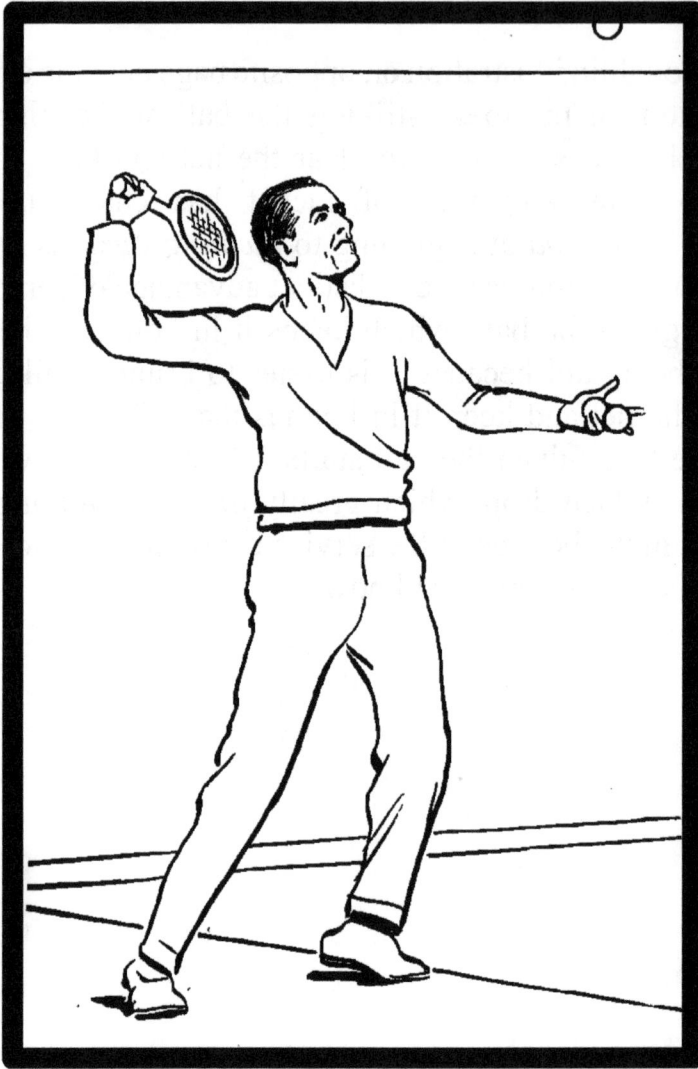

WILLIAM T. TILDEN…..In the act of tossing the ball
*Note how slight upward bend of the arm. Ball has been tossed into air by flick of the wrist. Only **consistent** method*

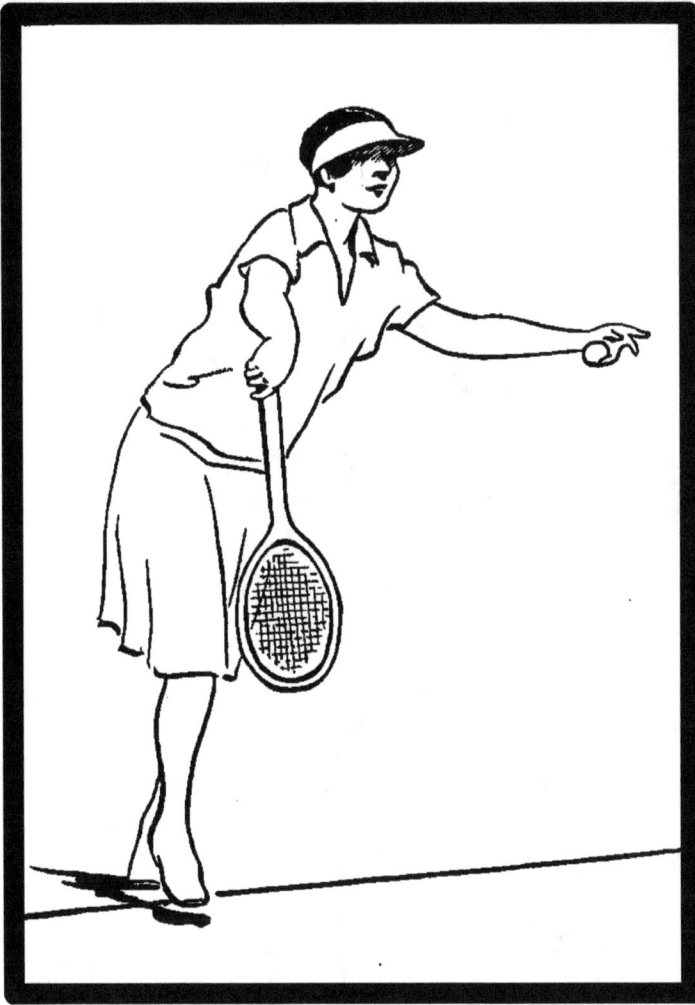

HELEN WILLS….. Finishes on the left side
She has the best service among the best women tennis player in the
world.

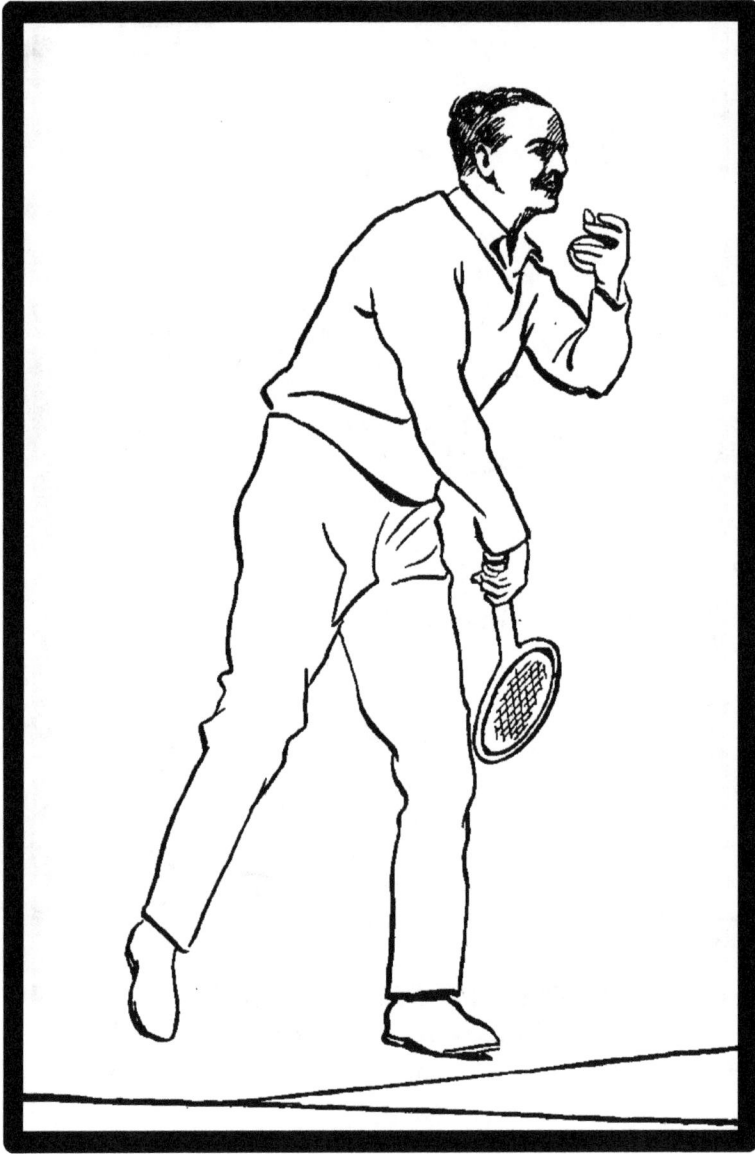

WILLIAM JOHNSTON

Note finishes on the left side of the body. The former champion throws
the ball toward the right shoulder, slightly in front of the body.

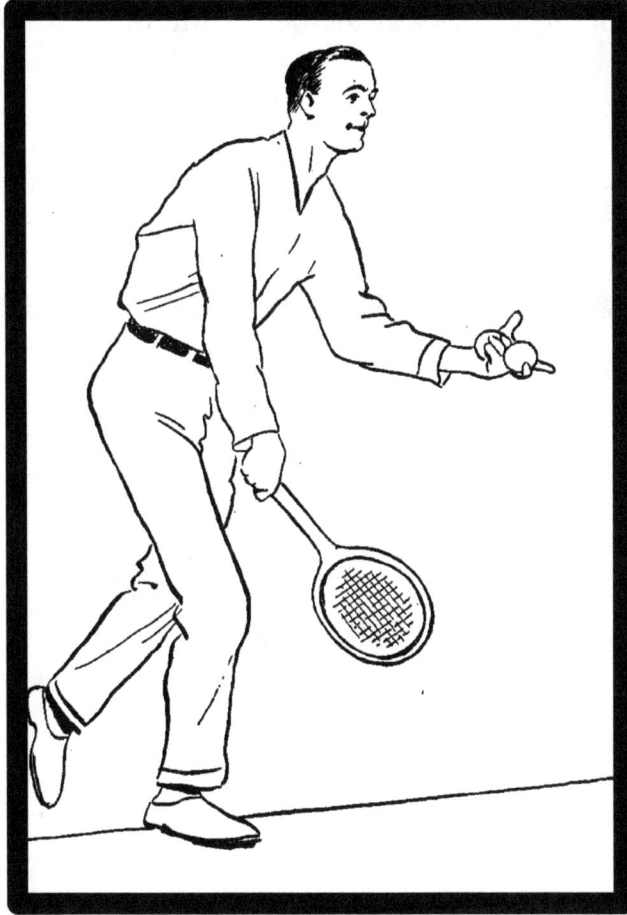

TILDEN'S..... Finish on his left side, weight forward.

WEIGHT

The transfer of weight into the stroke is what gives it additional power.

It is a well-known fact that there is no power in the punch of a pugilist if the punch is delivered when he is falling back or gliding away. Hit the tennis ball as though you intended to advance into the net and not to retreat to the backstop nor glide away to the sidestop.

The weight should be back at the beginning of the stroke and forward at the finish.

In order to get your weight into the shot it is necessary to strike the ball right at your side in the drive, not out in front nor too far behind. Therefore, it is better to run more or less directly at your ball and then sidestep it, rather than to run in circles and be continually reaching for the ball.

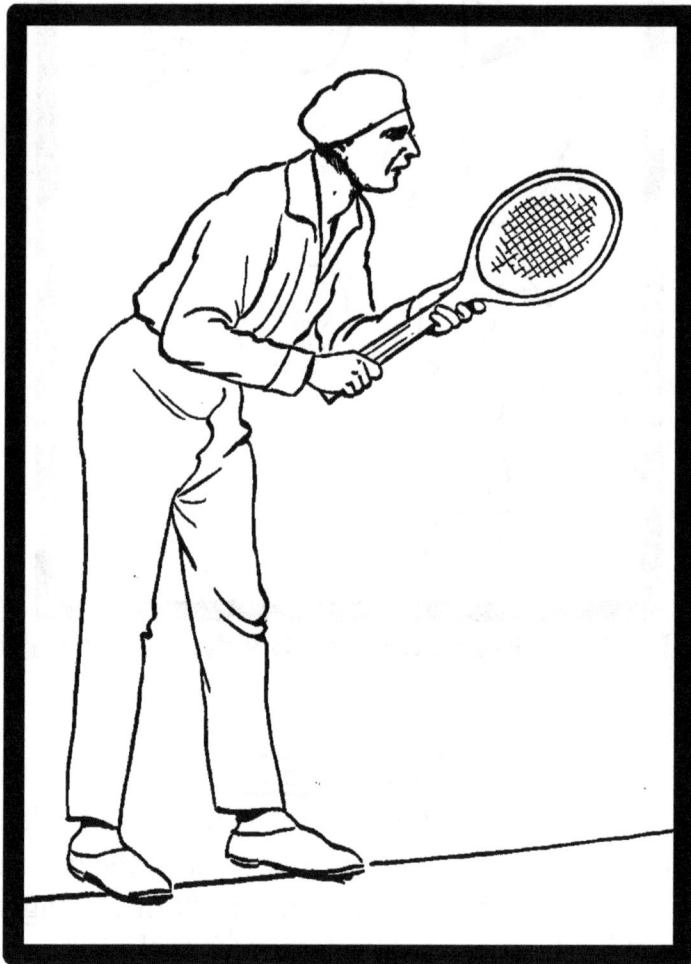

JEAN BOROTRA

154

Note on opposite page, the easy, alert, waiting-to-receive-service of this well-known French player. He has his forearm grip, but it is merely a matter of preference which grip you assume.

Borotra's feet are on the baseline, a couple of feet from the sideline. This is the position the quick-moving, keen-eyed Frenchmen take to return the swiftest service, for they strike the ball as it rises.

Only the most skillful can risk standing in so close. I recommend a position at least a couple of feet behind the base line, and often further back, to receive the swift first service, moving in closer for the slower second service.

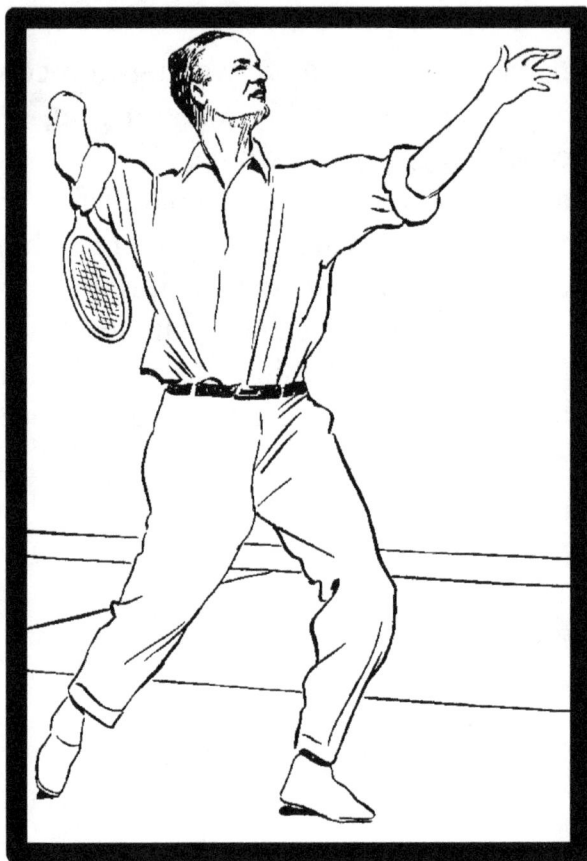

WILLIAM JOHNSTON……. Prepared
In taking overhead smash- racket back long before arrival of ball.

OVERHEAD SMASH

The smashing of a lob while it is still high in the air is one of the most beautiful and exhilarating shots in tennis. It is played with a service grip and is brought down just as you would bring your service down.

The principal mistake which a poor overhead player makes is in not getting *under* the ball.

Your position is the same as if you were playing baseball and were running to catch a fly. You would not attempt to catch it out in front of you nor too far behind, but you would run to a position *directly under* the ball. So it is with the smash.

You should jump into the air when possible, in order to strike the ball at the very top of your extended reach, for the higher you can contact the ball the more forcibly you can bring it down into your opponent's court.

If you are netting your overheads, it is probable that you are getting them too far in front of you.

If you are sending them out of court, then you are probably letting them get too low, so that you cannot get over them in order to smash them down.

If the high smash comes to your backhand side, and it is high enough in the air so that you have time to maneuver into position to smash from the forehand side, by all means do so, because only a few extraordinary players can smash with power or accuracy from the backhand side.

Often a sharply angled, cleverly placed smash will score more readily than the hard smash to the back court.

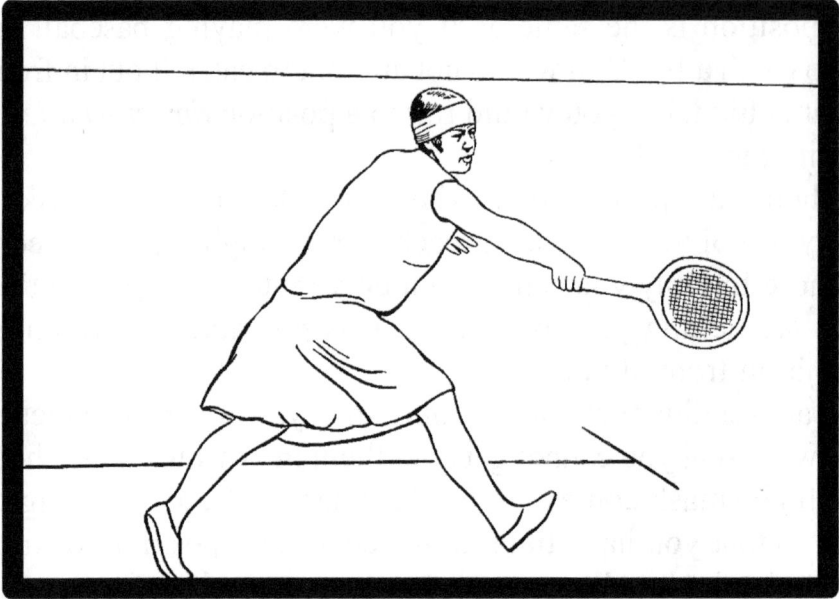

MOLLA MALLORY……. *Returns a backhand from near net*
Molla's middle name is "activity". She goes for everything.

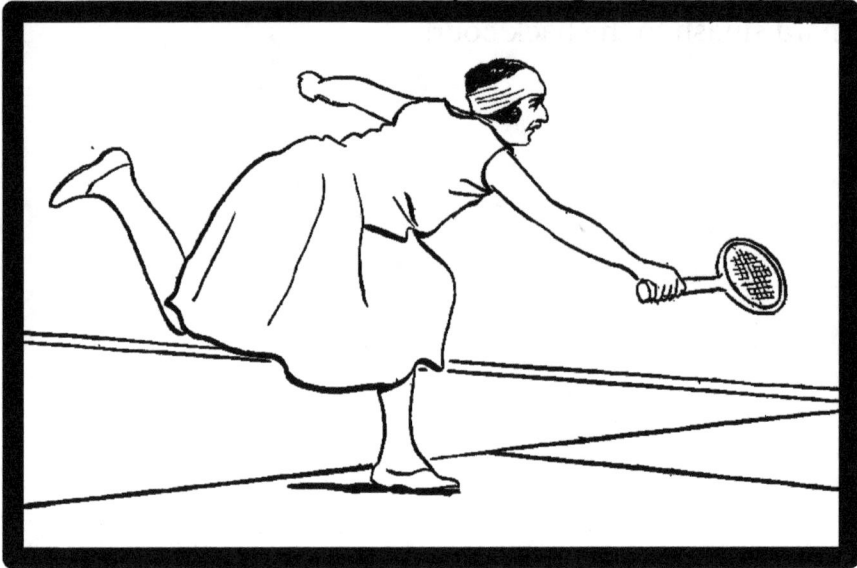

SUZANNE LENGLEN…..Gets down to a low volley.

THE VOLLEY

The volley is a ball played before it touches the court at a position close to the net. A large gesture is not made for the volley, as in the drive, just a short stroke, but a stroke nevertheless. The correct volley grip is the same as for the backhand.

It is most important to keep the head of the racket higher than, or as high as, the wrist, which necessitates your getting down to your shots, so low often that one knee touches the court.

Direct the ball with a *definite* forward finish. There is little or no backswing necessary, but it is important to follow through.

When one is at the net with the back court unprotected, then one must not send a weak return off the volley, for it gives your opponent the opportunity to pass you or to lob over your head.

Whenever possible, step forward to meet your volley rather than wait for it to come to you.

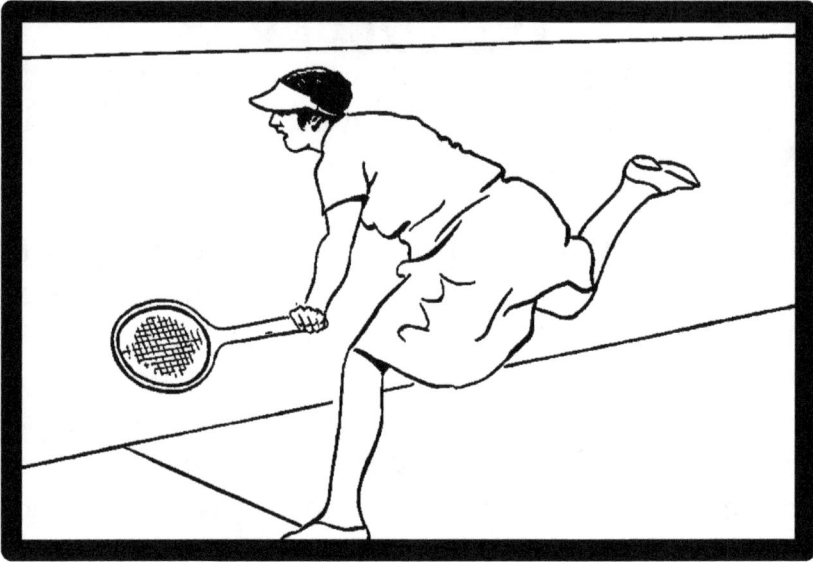

HELEN WILLS…. Stepping lively.

Tennis is a game of activity. You must be ready- willing- and capable of moving fast- to play tennis well.

It is important to volley the ball before it has dropped below the top of the net is possible.

Deliberation

To volley accurately you must be deliberate, just as in making your ground strokes.

You will say: "How can we be deliberate when the balls are flying at us like shots out of a gun?" Still, it always seems possible that the quick-thinking and fast-moving player gets to the ball so quickly that he can take that little extra time to deliberate, even though it may be a split second.

This is very conspicuous in the volleys of Vincent Richards. He seldom if ever gives the impression of being hurried. In fact, one feels that he is never going to hit the ball.

Undoubtedly it is this deliberation which gives him poise and such phenomenal control at the net.

Hurry to position but take your time making your strokes. Too many players lag on the footwork and hurry their strokes.

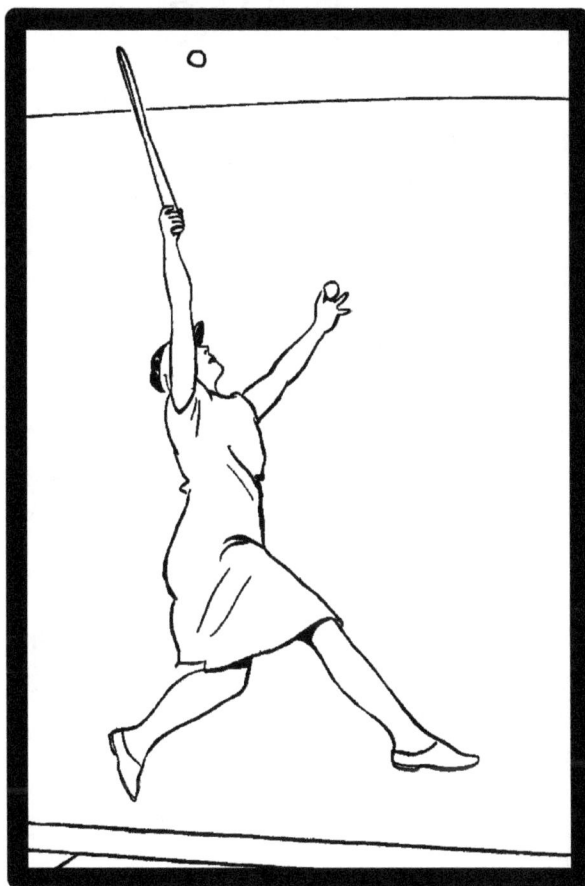

HELEN WILLS…..Goes up after a high one.
If you can jump, you may play closer to the net without fear of being lobbed over. The higher you can reach the ball the easier you can bring it down.

THE HIGH LOB

A high lob is harder to "kill" than a low lob because a high lob drops straighter down and faster on account of the greater drag of the forces of gravity. It is advisable to play

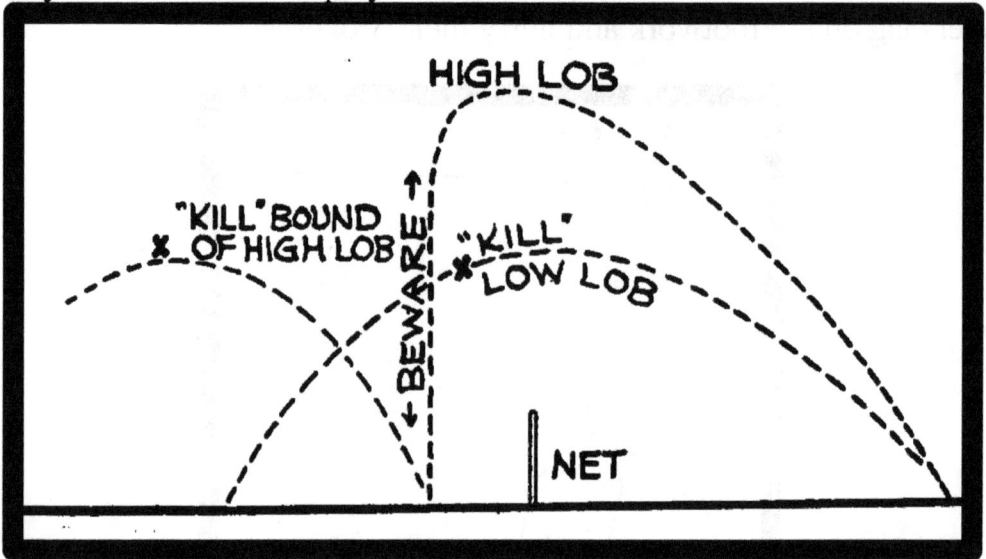

it back defensively, or let it bound, and then you have a ball much like a low lob, which you can smash with safety.

Since it is harder to "kill" a high lob, when you are lobbing in self-defense, *start your lob high*. Then, if it should drop short in your opponent's court, you are in less danger than if your lob was started low.

Sky is the limit for a defensive lob.

STRAIGHT-DOWN-THE-LINE SHOT

The shot down the line in singles in invaluable, both as a passing shot and to attack your opponent's weakness.

Be careful about the higher net.

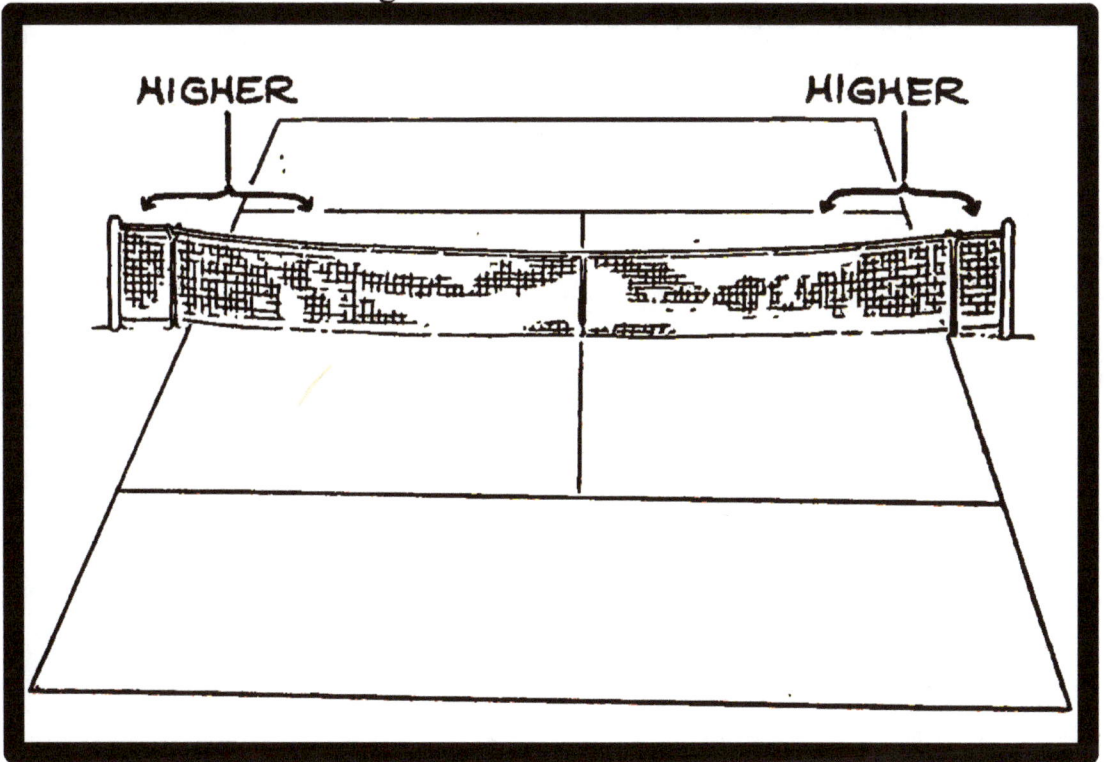

There is a very important consideration when playing the backhand shot straight down the line. If the ball you are planning to return down the line has come to you in the form of a sharply angled *cross-court drive* from your opponent's racket, then be sure and *aim* your return a couple of feet *inside* the sideline rather than directly at the line.

The angle at which the ball meets your racket makes it curve to the outside and you will find many of these shots landing in the alley just outside the court.

If your opponent's return comes to you from only slightly off center in his court to slightly off center in your court, then you can afford to aim your return closer to the line.

It is easier to play a drive cross court than straight down the line, because net is higher at side lines.

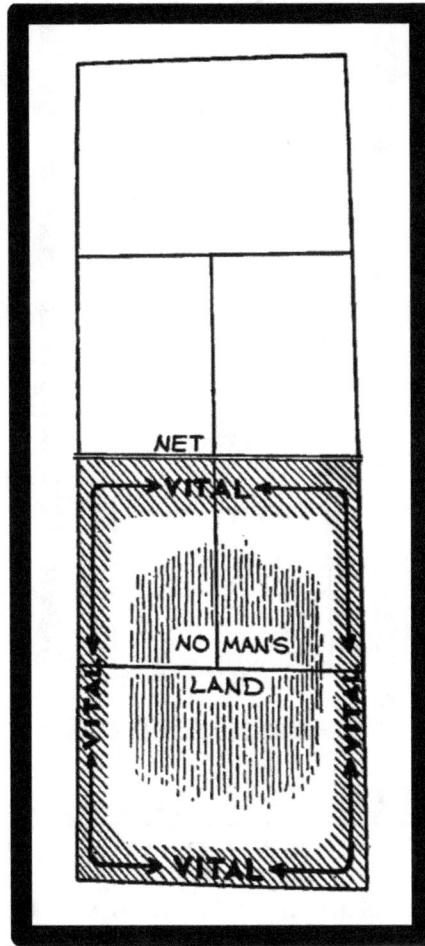

DESTINATION OF SHOT MORE IMPORTANT THAN SPEED

Suzanne Lenglen has pointed out the VITAL territory of her opponent's court more conspicuously than any other living tennis player.

Any shot not landing in the portion of the court marked "VITAL" is wasted, according to Suzanne.

"No Man's Land" is the territory to be avoided. Returns in this portion of the court, dealt with by an expert, will meet sudden death.

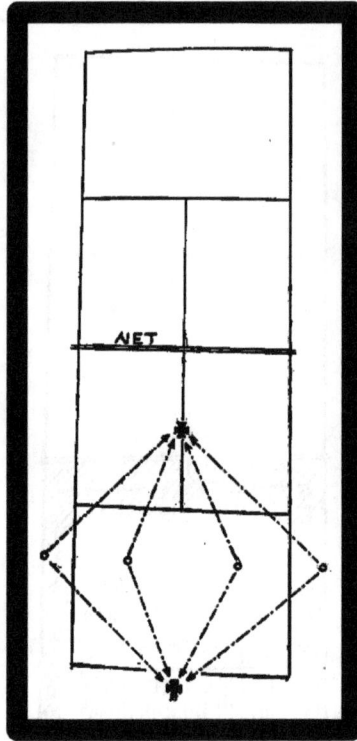

POSITION ON THE COURT IS ONE-THIRD THE BATTLE

In singles, when you return the ball from any point on or off the court (as indicated by the circles on the diagram), you must *immediately* return to a position behind the baseline at the center or go up to the net at the center (as indicated in the diagram by the crosses).

Do not wait to see your return land, but as soon as you make your return, recover your position at once.

This is absolutely essential to enable you to cover all points of your court successfully.

Your position should be *clear up* or *clear back* never halfway.

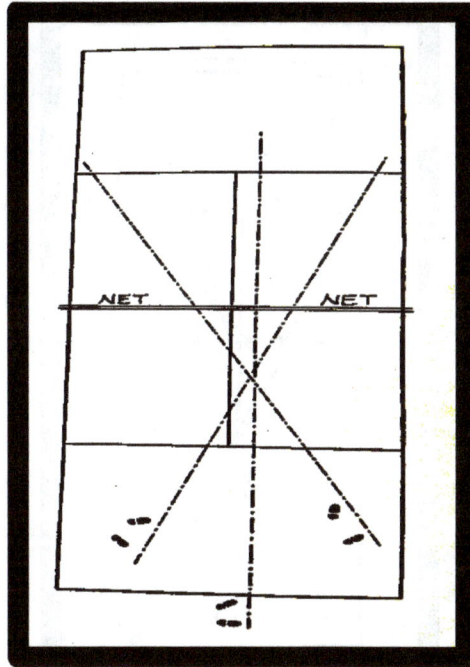

BODY PLACEMENT AN IMPORTANT FACTOR IN *BALL* PLACEMENT

The position of the body (shown in diagram by position of the feet) has a great deal to do with the placing of the drive.

The feet should be parallel with the line of flight.

This position of the body makes it possible for the finish of the follow-through to be in the direction you wish your ball to take.

The only disadvantage of this method is that, to a keen opponent, the position of your body "telegraphs" the destination of your shot and helps him anticipate your return.

Nevertheless, getting your ball to the spot is far more important than disguising your intention.

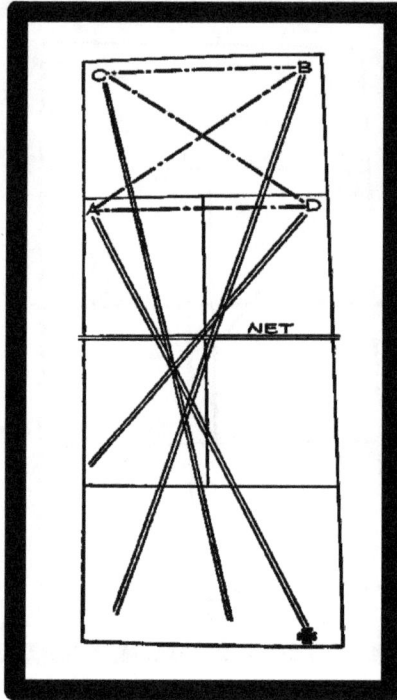

A SCHEDULE OF PLAYS

Suzanne Lenglen has a schedule of plays in a singles match. Regardless of where you place your return, Suzanne is so accurate that she can carry out her schedule, which is a combination of deep baseline drives alternated with a slower cross-court angle. It is in reality a *sequence* of plays which makes the most effective use of the VITAL territory.

You can readily see that her opponents are obliged to cover the maximum of court. Nor does Suzanne care if you anticipate and reach her returns, because the more you reach the more energy you expend, and her tactics are designed to exhaust you.

The broken lines indicate the way Suzanne's opponents must run as the result of her returns in sequence A—B—C—D.

STRENGTHEN A WEAKNESS. DO NOT PROTECT IT

Do not make a practice of running around your backhand and taking the ball on the forearm, because you will continually be out of position and have to cover a great deal more court. By protecting a weakness, you simply contribute to that weakness, and eventually you will meet a player who will make you play the game from your weak stroke.

If you are playing against a player who runs around the ball to avoid taking it on the backhand, place your first return well to his forearm court, thus drawing him to the right side of his court; then you can get the ball down to his backhand without trouble; whereas, if you just keep laying to his backhand continually, he can keep running around them.

"GETS" IN TENNIS

There are many occasions when you cannot get into position to take your stroke, but you must still try to return the ball.

These are the "gets" in tennis which thrill the gallery and make you the winner. Get the ball back any old way—both hands if necessary—only, *get it back*.

I have known good players who were the essence of grace when set for their return, yet when they were in difficulties, and there was no graceful way in which to extricate themselves, I have seen them return balls sitting on the court after a spoil, or on their knees, but they never ceased to try to keep the ball in play.

THE DROP SHOT

The drop shot is usually played with a very short grip; that is, the hand is slipped up the handle and the ball popped over the net with a push stroke. Change of grip and the position of the racket, however, is apt to "Telegraph" the shot to an opponent.

Played to just clear the net and drop as closely as possible to it, the drop shot is difficult to control. It is easier to play it at an angle to one side or the other rather than straight over the net. It is dangerous if it does not drop very near the net, which always involves the risk of netting; so, therefore, only under exceptional occasions do you find it used. When an opponent is far behind the baseline and you have an easy mid-court return, drop it just over the net. Should your opponent reach this shot, your logical next return is a lob over his head.

CHANGE OF PACE AND ANGLES

The finesse of tennis requires that the player control a short slow shot as well as those played swiftly to the back line. If you can only do one or two things, then your opponent knows what to expect and is prepared.

If you occasionally play a soft drop shot or slow-angled drive just over the net, your opponent dare not play too far behind the baseline, for fear of the short one; therefore, you keep him guessing. The most difficult running on the tennis court is up to the net and back to the position behind the baseline, not from side to side of the back court.

The distance from a yard back of the baseline to the net is farther than from side to side, and after running up you must retreat backwards, which is exhausting. So, if you can control the drop shot and sharp angles you can draw your opponent up and back.

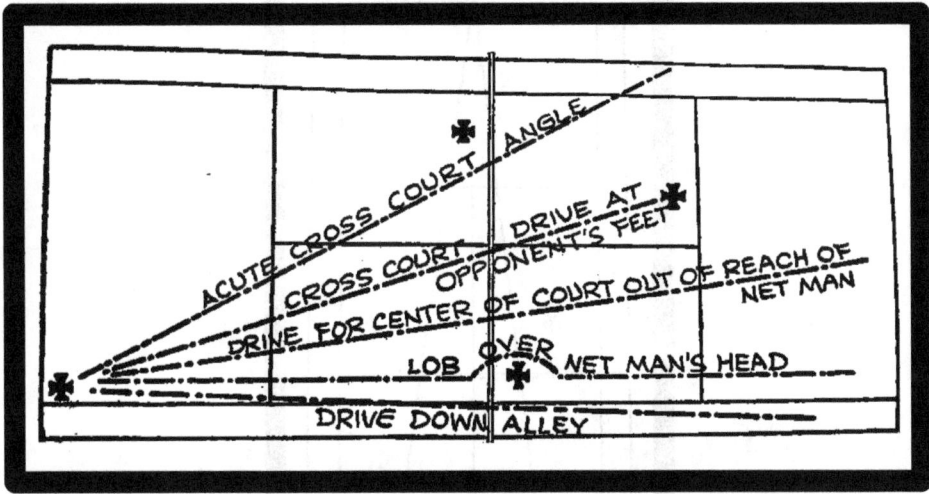

FIVE WAYS TO REPLY TO SERVICE IN DOUBLES

1. Cross-court drive aimed at the feet of advancing opponent is the one shot most frequently used. (Because it is the least dangerous.)

2. Lob over net man's head. (Used to force an opponent away from the net.)

3. Acute cross-court angle. (Passing shot.)

4. Drive for center of the court, just out of the reach of net man. (Mixes up your opponents' teamwork.)

5. Drive down the alley. (Useful in keeping the net man from poaching.)

Spreading the fingers slightly up the handle of the racket helps give control—BUT—*practice, practice, practice* of the strokes is the thing which contributes MOST to control.

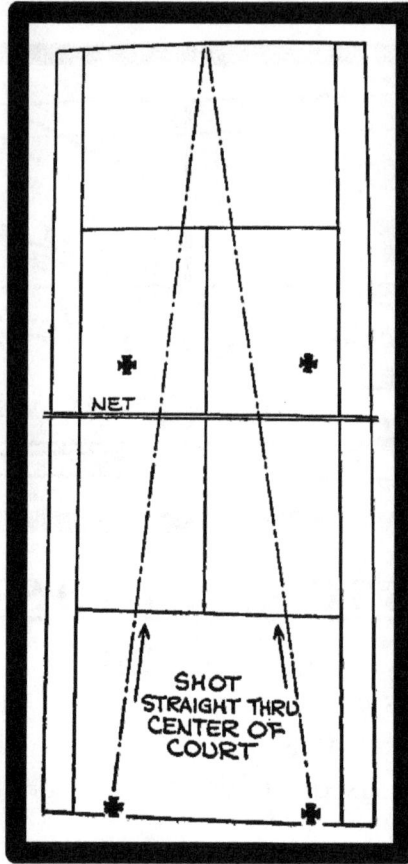

STRATEGY OF SHOT THROUGH CENTER

The shot straight through the center of the court is a fine shot in doubles. It mixes up the opponents' teamwork. The slight hesitation as to who shall take the ball often proves fatal.

Each team should make a point of deciding which should take the ball, and the things which should influence them, and which usually decides the point is leaving it with the man playing left court and covering center balls on his forearm; or there are occasions when it is best that the man who has made the last return be allowed to follow up the play. Or, if one is hopelessly out of position, then the partner must take the ball regardless. You can see why the shot through the center of the court is apt to be confusing.

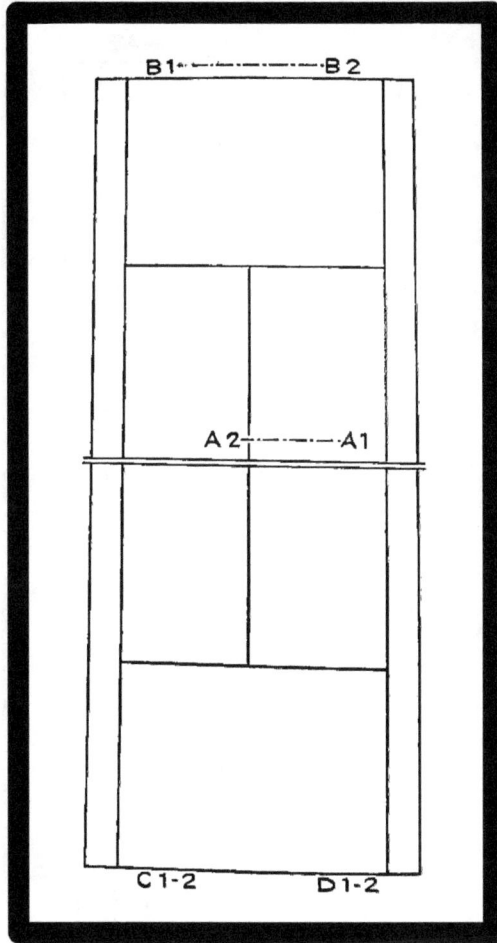

POACHING

If you poach in tennis at the net and have crossed over to your partner's side as in the case of A to position No. 2 in the diagram, you must *stay* over, and your partner takes the other side in his No. 2 position.

Should you switch back and forth from one side of the net to the other, your partner will be completely demoralized, not knowing which side to take.

The only excuse for you to cross the second time is for an easy "kill", which should end the point.

B1 A3

B 2·3

A

OVER

A1 A2

C3 D3

LOB

C1-2 D1-2

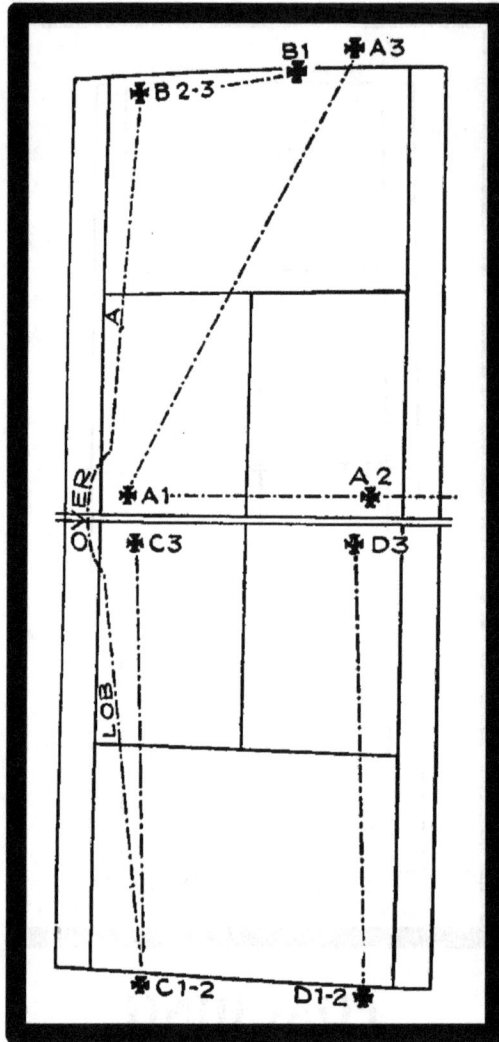

DOUBLES FORMATION

A, *B*, *C*, and *D*'s first position finds *B* serving. *C* lobs over *A*'s head; both *C* and *D* remain in their first position in the back court. *A* must cross over to his second position at the net, while his partner *B* retrieves the ball. Should *C* and *D* decided to come to the net in their position No. 3, then *A* must come back to the back court, to his position No. 3, with is partner *B* retrieving the ball in his position Nos. 2 and 3. This change will never leave any part of the court unprotected.

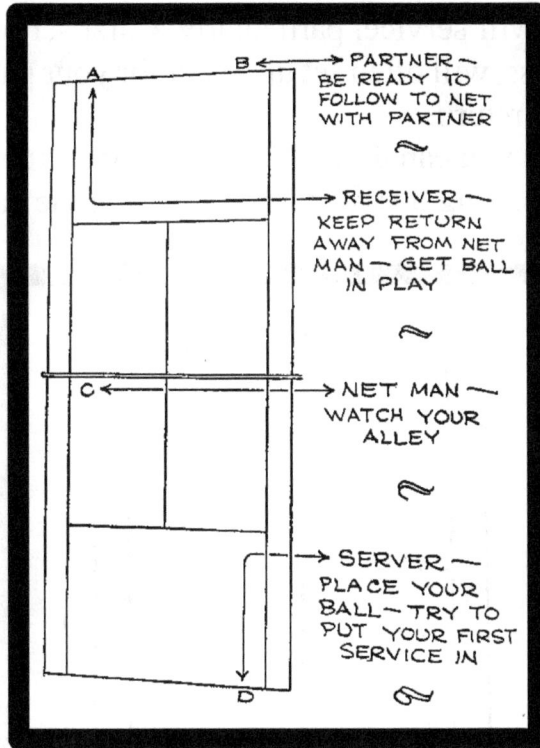

A
B ←
→ PARTNER ~
BE READY TO
FOLLOW TO NET
WITH PARTNER
~

→ RECEIVER ~
KEEP RETURN
AWAY FROM NET
MAN ~ GET BALL
IN PLAY
~

C ←
→ NET MAN ~
WATCH YOUR
ALLEY
~

→ SERVER ~
PLACE YOUR
BALL ~ TRY TO
PUT YOUR FIRST
SERVICE IN
~

D

DOUBLES TACTICS

On the opposite and two following pages are diagrams in which I have tried to impart some doubles advice.

The *Doubles* game s very different from the *Singles* game. In doubles you must consider your partner at every turn and direct your play with the idea of setting up shots for him.

For example, if you place a sharp crosscourt angle at your opponent's feet as he advances to the net, he will be obliged to lift the ball to clear the net, and very often your partner can pounce upon it for a "kill".

Your partner will probably get the applause for the kill, but understanding tennis fans will give you credit for the setup.

A well-placed swift service, particularly a first service, placed to your opponent's weakness, will often set up a shot for your partner, because you have forced a weak return.

However, just as you can give your partner opportunities, you can also get him in bad, by putting up weak lobs or getting the ball

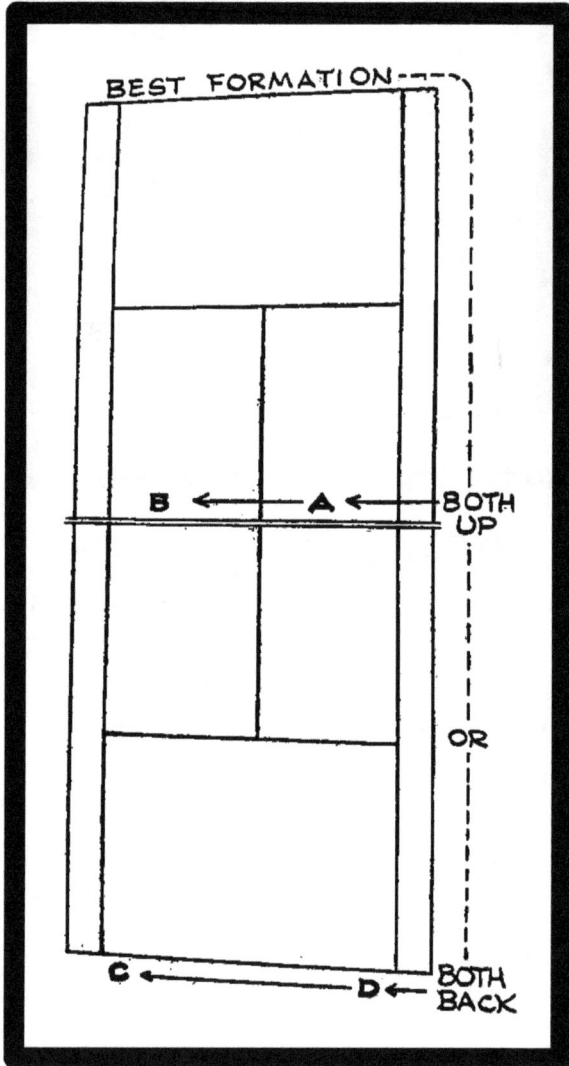

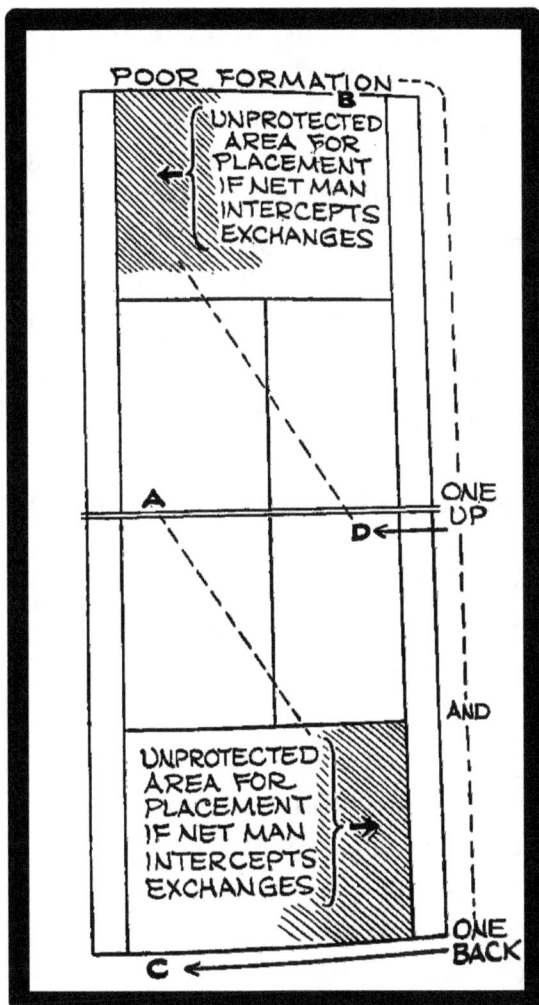

POOR FORMATION

B
UNPROTECTED AREA FOR PLACEMENT IF NET MAN INTERCEPTS EXCHANGES

A

D

ONE UP

AND

UNPROTECTED AREA FOR PLACEMENT IF NET MAN INTERCEPTS EXCHANGES

C

ONE BACK

into the net man's hands, on the return of service in particular. Again, your opponents can all but annihilate your partner, if you put over an easy lollypop second service.

Doubles take teamwork and tact. You should arrange for the stronger player to take left court, because the deciding points are played in this court. Also, the center territory comes on the forearm of the left court player. Have your understanding before you start play, so that you are not incessantly giving advice during play.

If your partner starts badly, try and forget him and concentrate on bringing up the standard of your own play. If you play well, it will greatly assist him in getting straightened out; whereas, if you worry over him, your own game and his, too, are doomed.

When you are at the net, watch your alley, because if your opponent's pass you down the alley, the point is lost, for it is nearly impossible for your partner to retrieve the ball. There is nothing so discouraging to your partner as to have you continually passed down the alley.

Try and get back under your own lobs. Your partner can advance to the net with far greater confidence if he does not have to back you up. It is far less confusing, too, in teamwork. But, if a lob is sent over your head, and your partner must go for it, then you must take the other side of the court, so that you leave no part of your court unprotected.

It is more important in doubles to get your first service in play than it is in singles.

In doubles you are continually trying to make openings to win your point, not by speed as much as by placement.

Get the ball in play off the service and do not take too many chances slamming the ball.

In singles you try for more speed and play the straight-down-the-line shots, while in doubles you are obliged to play the crosscourt drives most of the time and try for safe placements.

Lastly—and certainly not the least today—winning doubles means possession of the net. Get there as quickly as you can and if your opponents are in possession, try the tactics which will force them back. Here is where the lob comes into its own.

CAN WOMEN PLAY AT THE NET EFFECTIVELY IN SINGLES?

The majority of experts today think it is practically impossible for women to play the net in singles, because it requires speed of foot and a great deal of stamina, as they must get in quickly so as to cut off their opponent's return at a sharp angle and at the same time be agile enough to get back under a lob.

This up-and-back moving on the tennis court is more exhausting than a back-and-forth moving across the baseline.

The player who ventures to the net must anticipate in order to intercept the opponent's effort to pass her. Then deal with the return decisively, so as to end the point at once, or the net position is not for her.

In *doubles*, playing at the net is imperative and much easier. You have far less court to cover because you have the help of a partner. Possession of the net in doubles is nine-tenths of the battle, but it is risky in singles.

HOW AND WHEN TO ADVANCE TO THE NET IN SINGLES

If you find that you can win points by coming to the net in singles—though I warn you it is dangerous, for you are "fighting close in" —you must prepare for your advance and not just rush in indiscreetly.

Always, the ball you may follow to the net *must* be deep in your opponent's back court. It is suicide to advance to the net on a ball which is mid-court, for it is simple—for even an average player—to pass you.

There is a difference of opinion as to whether it is better to play the ball deep in the center of your opponent's back court—on the theory that they can only pass you with a sharp angle, which is in danger of landing out of court—or whether it is better to advance to the net on a deep shot to the corners of your opponent's back court. The latter gives him a long, though narrow, expanse of court down the side lines to play his passing shot. It gives to the net player, however, a large, unprotected part of his opponent's court into which he may return the volley with a much better chance to win the point outright.

Personally, I prefer the deep shot to the corner to prepare for the net, watching closely the shot straight down the line. The best corner of the court, in nine cases out of ten, is the backhand corner of your opponent's court, for the return is not apt to be so severe, and as a result easier to return.

Vincent Richards relies upon the center theory for his advance to the net, while William Johnston prefers the deep corners. There is merit in both.

However, you may be the most brilliant volleyer in the world, but if your ground strokes are not sound enough to place the ball properly to prepare for the advance, then you cannot play the net in singles.

<u>START AND FINISH PSYCHOLOGY</u>

Which is more vital in a tennis match, a good start or a fine finish?

It is difficult to say when it depends so much on the temperament of the individual, for there are players who will become demoralized if their opponents start well and acquire a considerable lead against them, and there are others who are at their best when they are behind.

It never makes any difference to William Tilden if his opponent defeats him 6-0 the first set. Tilden can go on to victory. He even seems to enjoy being behind and making his dramatic finish. I have seen him many times within a point of defeat and till win. In fact, I feel that Tilden seldom tries to put forth his best efforts in the preliminary games.

Henri Cochet is a bad starter. Not from indifference but because he has trouble getting the range of the court and his delicate timing of the ball under control in the first stages. He has, luckily for him, good nerve and self-confidence. His finish is usually brilliant. He is, however, too extreme in both directions, letting himself in for tremendous uphill fights, too often late, with his brilliance.

Mrs. Jessup and Eleanor Goss, former members of the American Wightman Cup team, are very good starters and poor finishers.

This is the main reason why they have threatened to win, but have never succeeded in winning, the national championship.

The good finisher, as a rule, has an infinitely better opportunity to win than the good starter who weakens toward the end of his match, but the tennis-wise players, like Rene Lacoste, Helen Wills and Suzanne Lenglen, seem to strike the happy medium, starting and finishing with equal dash.

VICTORY IS A FAST PACEMAKER

Once players could go to big luncheons, eat plentifully, return to the court and win, in spite of being stogy and slow. The days when a good forearm drive, and noting much else, was sufficient.

Today *Victory* is a fast pacemaker. The winner must be "on his toes" every moment, fit and in good form. It means absolute concentration. It means sacrifice and hard work. Other interests to a degree are subordinated.

You cannot set your own pace. Like the contestants in the six-day cycle races, you must "sprint" when the other fellow does or lose out. A short absence from actual competition may mean that even though you have not lost ground, your opponents have improved while you were standing still.

Tennis is not standing still, and what was good enough yesterday may not be good enough to win from the same player tomorrow.

To win consistently one must almost cease to be an individual and become a force in the one game in which he is looking for victory.

FIGHTING SPIRIT

"And he is dead who will not fight."

I wonder sometimes if fighting spirit can be cultivated? Someone laughed heartily at me once when I said, "So-and-So has cultivated a sense of humor."

The claim was that people are born with a sense of humor. If so, perhaps champions are born with a will-to-win spirit, and if they are not so equipped at birth they many never acquire it.

I am not so pessimistic. I believe that at least a fairly workable substitute can be acquired by perseverance and mental training. Then, too, it may be there dormant but never aroused.

At any rate, it is in its essence a spirit which never says die; which plugs when matches seem lost; consistent concentration and belief in one's self.

All thoughts of failure must be put out of mind—*Mental Uncertainty Definitely Causes Shaky and Uncertain Muscular Co-ordination.*

There are hundreds of thrilling incidences when victory has been snatched from defeat.

In 1927, at Wimbledon, "Big Bill" Tilden led two sets to one and 5-1 in the fourth set. He needed only one game for the match when his opponent, Henri Cochet, the brilliant young Frenchman, staged what is considered one of the most spectacular and disconcerting upsets in tennis history. Cochet won this match from an utterly confused Tilden.

It seemed scarcely possible for this to happen to a player of Tilden's worldwide experience. It can happen to anyone, and you can someday be the hero of such a victory if you have the nerve, fight and self-confidence. Also, you may be victim.

<u>THE WINNING SYSTEM</u>

Begins and ends with accuracy and control.
Acquired by an intelligent understanding and thorough knowledge of the fundamentals.

<u>Then Practice, Practice, Practice</u>

Conservation of your energy while exhausting your opponent.
By a system of plays which not only run your opponent back and forth on the baseline, but also up and back from the net.

Anticipation
Study your opponent's habit of making fixed replies.
Study their ways of "telegraphing" advance information.
Be alert and ready to move on the ball.

Minimize your errors
By sacrificing speed for accuracy.
By clearing the net well on each return.
Get the ball in play off the service.

Footwork

Do not stand flatfooted; balance lightly and be ready to move in any direction.

Turn sideways for your deep strokes.

After each stroke recover your position immediately, either back behind the baseline or up to the net.

Timing

Be so quick into position that you can be deliberate in making your stroke.

Bombard your opponent's weakness

Fight with self-confidence and a determination to win, but Play Fair.

THE POWER OF CONCENTRATION

Recently, I read an article by a very famous woman journalist who had interviewed hundreds of successful men. She was asked if there was any one characteristic which was common to all. It was not a question she could answer offhand. She gave it deep thought and her conclusion was that these men did have one thing in common. That was *power of concentration*, to a far greater degree than the average man.

If there is any common ground upon which all successful athletes tread, it is upon the ground charged with a high degree of concentration.

They may be tall or short, dark or fair, but all possess, to a greater degree than the average human, that power of concentration.

SELECTING THE RACKET

The grip should not be too large for the hand. For a woman, 4 ½ to 4 ¾ inches is the average size of the grip. A man can use one larger but should not have over a 5-inch grip. The tendency is toward smaller grips. A large grip tires the hand and there is no feel to the racket that clogs the palm.

The weight of a racket for a woman should be from 12½ to 13½ ounces. Neither under nor over these weights. The average weight for men should be from 13 to 14 ounces. For both men and women I believe in an even balance. The racket then feels like an extension of the arm, and though the weight is there, one is not conscious of it.

A light racket is easier to handle, especially at the net, but one too light requires extra exertion from the back court on ground strokes, and therefore increases the difficulties in timing the ball.

THE MODEL GAME

I am incorporating in this book extracts from an article which I wrote for "The Saturday Evening Post", immediately following a four months' tour with Suzanne Lenglen, during which time I opposed her in forty singles matches and many more doubles matches.

The extracts describe "A Tennis Game" which I believe is the best pattern for any aspiring tennis enthusiast, either man or woman. It is as nearly foolproof as the combined heads of many past masters and an apt pupil can make the game. You cannot do better than to copy it until you feel that you can improve it.

In all the years I have played the game, I realize now that I had overlooked the simplest rudiments of tennis, which are the foundation of Suzanne's games.

She is not, as nearly everyone supposes, a prodigy at all. She is a product of intelligent coaching, persistent practice and keen observation. Of course, she has unusual speed of foot and a rare tennis mind, but I have known many women players who had such qualities but never scaled the heights that Suzanne has. In natural ability May Sutton Bundy was the equal of Suzanne, but like the rest of us, she did not have the same quality of coaching and systematic training in technic.

Suzanne has a purpose in every move she makes. Her accuracy can hardly be improved on. Having the necessary control of her shots, she can play a crafty game which allows her to conserve her energy while forcing her opponent to wear herself out.

Although she can, if she wishes, drive with as much power as most men, she rarely does so, for, as she explains, power is gained at the sacrifice of accuracy, and her game is based on perfect control. Most players try to win on placements. Suzanne rarely tries a placement until she has maneuvered you out of position or forced a weak return. But an examination of the point score of most of her matches, particularly important matches, shows that she usually relies on the simple process of keeping the ball in play until her opponent makes an error.

She can volley better than any woman I have seen, but she seldom goes to the net unless drawn there. Lenglen, in fact, has perfected every stroke. There **is** not, in my opinion, any woman who compares with her in any way, with the possible exception that Helen Wills strokes with greater severity.

Ninety-nine players out of a hundred, including the men, drive as closely as possible to the top of the net, but Suzanne invariably clears the net by a good foot. A hard-driven ball that clears the net by a scant inch is no more effective than Suzanne's ball that clears it well. It is the destination of the ball that is important, and the player who tries to skin the net on most of his returns will send a large portion of them into the net.

COVERING GROUND

"What good is a brilliant thought behind the ball which ends in the net?" asks Suzanne. Obviously, the answer is: "No good." She rarely loses her points by netting, and in many of her hardest matches the point score will show not more than half a dozen nets, compared with twenty or thirty for nearly any capable player you can mention.

Next to clearing the net, Suzanne's basic strategy is to conserve her energy and at the same time to wear out her opponent. In a sense, every return she makes is to the point farthest removed from the previous one, so that you cover the maximum distance. With many players, the execution of this strategy finds expression in drives first to the right-hand corner of the court, then to the left or backhand, corner. They keep an opponent running back and forth with the monotonous regularity of a pendulum.

Suzanne does not rely upon making you run across the backline. She can shorten her drives and place them at acute angles to the sidelines. Thus you are forced to advance to the net and retreat again to the baseline, which means that one is forced to cover a maximum of court, both up and back, as well as from side to side.

The up-and-back running is the most exhausting, for one does not usually turn one's back to the opponent but retreats backward.

Suzanne can effectively carry on a campaign of wearing down her opponent, because she can not only keep the ball in play but has the accuracy to place the ball constantly to the proper portion of her opponent's court to force her to do the running.

She makes players run rapidly and incessantly to reach her returns, while she appears to be waiting for their returns when the ball arrives. This is due to her having been drilled in what the logical return will be from her opponent's racket, plus her own keen observation of the tendency of her opponent to make certain fixed replies.

THE OPPONENT'S GAME UNDER CONTROL

Tennis critics are apt to dismiss Suzanne's marvelous ability always to be in position, waiting, by calling it uncanny anticipation and marvelous speed of foot. It is more than that. I maintain that other players have those qualities. I may say—I hope with modesty—that I myself have possessed anticipation and a good deal of fleetness, but I was never drilled from childhood in what the logical and almost invariable results of certain definite plays will be.

No player in the world, except Norman Brookes of Australia, in my opinion, has had such control over his opponent's game as has Suzanne. She can make you play into her hands. She can play you out of position in spite of any and everything you may try to do to avoid it. She can make three or four plays and tell you where she will end her point. Just as Willie Hoppe can tell you in advance of three of four plays the exact relative position in which the three billiard balls will stand, or just as John McGraw can tell you in advance the position of his men on base as the result of, say, a single, a sacrifice and a two-bagger.

Suzanne has been drilled in these sequences of plays, in a schedule of shots, and she has several combination s at her command. She is not a genius born but a genius made. It is the hard work she has done to perfect her technic, the research and systematic study of every type of player combined, which has made of her game a perfect machine, recognized, I believe, by the greatest players, both men and women, as the pattern for future development in tennis.

Rene Lacoste, more than any of the Frenchmen, has studied Suzanne and used her tactics. He is now the champion of America, the first foreigner in twenty years

to hold our title. He will, I believe, continue his success, for his game is grounded on sound technic and basic principles which are bound to succeed.

I shall state again briefly the things Suzanne has been taught about tennis which have done more to make her great than all her natural ability: To practice, practice, practice until she could control the ball well enough to play it from any position in her own court to any portion of her opponent's court; the absolutely essential five-finger exercises. No one is born with that skill. It comes from constantly doing the same thing over and over. The result is control.

Next, Suzanne was taught to put that control into use. She received the concentrated, predigested, tried, perfected and finally combined methods of the then best players in the wide world, such as Brookes and Wilding of Australia, Norris Williams of America, and the Dohertys of England. The best methods included the holding of the racket and the making of the strokes, as well as the best direction and destination of the shots.

Suzanne has told me that the backhand was very difficult for her to learn. It was entirely due to her father's persistent and insistent demands amid tears and scenes that she learned to make this stroke correctly. It is now the best executed of all her strokes.

Suzanne was schooled in tactics, just as our West Pointers are drilled and drilled in what is and what is not good soldiery. With the, just as with Suzanne, we are apt to confuse training which has become second nature with inherent genius. If a general makes a crafty move at exactly the right moment, to break up the enemy's defense, is it something new or an old method opportunely used?

Further, Suzanne was taught to minimize her errors. The same good advice has been given to many a poker player out of luck: "Minimize your losses."

SACRIFICING THE SPECTACULAR

One very simple thing she was taught and which her strokes were adapted to accomplish was to clear the net. Strangely enough, this is a simple thing which is as much neglected in tennis by very good players as looking at the golf ball until you have hit it is neglected in golf.

Another very effective way that Suzanne minimizes her errors is by not trying to make a kill on her opponent's difficult shots; she tries merely to return the ball safely. Then she does not herself hit any harder than is necessary to score the point.

There is a fiction that her father was accustomed to spreading a pocket handkerchief on the court and keeping Suzanne at practice until she was able to hit the target four times out of five.

Suzanne laughingly denies the legend. Her target was the vital area of the court adjacent to the sidelines.

Drives that do not reach a spot within this vital territory of her opponent's court are wasted, according to Suzanne.

I discovered that most of our crowds were surprised that Suzanne's game was soft—that she did not have a tremendous punch in her stroking. She sacrifices speed to gain in accuracy, and none can dispute that the results have justified her course. This method of play, however, frequently develops uninteresting tennis, but it is uninteresting only in the same sense that an efficient workman is. A baseball pitcher who strikes out he opposing batters or causes them to hit weakly to the fielders is making baseball uninteresting, or at least dulls its spectacular features, but he is a good pitcher.

So it is with Suzanne. Only one who is playing against her, or an expert, can see her delicate workmanship. For the most part she appears to be hitting lightly. But I assure you that her soft balls are most difficult to return cleanly. At times they appear almost to float over the net, but as you set about confidently to kill them something goes wrong. Your returns find the net or drift over the lines.

CHARACTERISTICS OF PLAY

That happens because the ball carries unsuspected pace or spin slyly imparted to it by Suzanne. The most subtle feature of her game is a change of pace—that elusive quality that Red Grange carries to the football field. A tackler gauges his speed and launches himself headlong as Grange, but usually he has passed the spot at which the tackler aimed or has not yet arrived. This disconcerting effect he achieves by increasing or decreasing his speed. But he does it almost imperceptibly, and the tackler does not suspect what has happened, until Grange glides by untouched.

The Greatest
Woman's Racket
Ever Made—

The

MARY K. BROWNE

Top-Flite

Model

$15

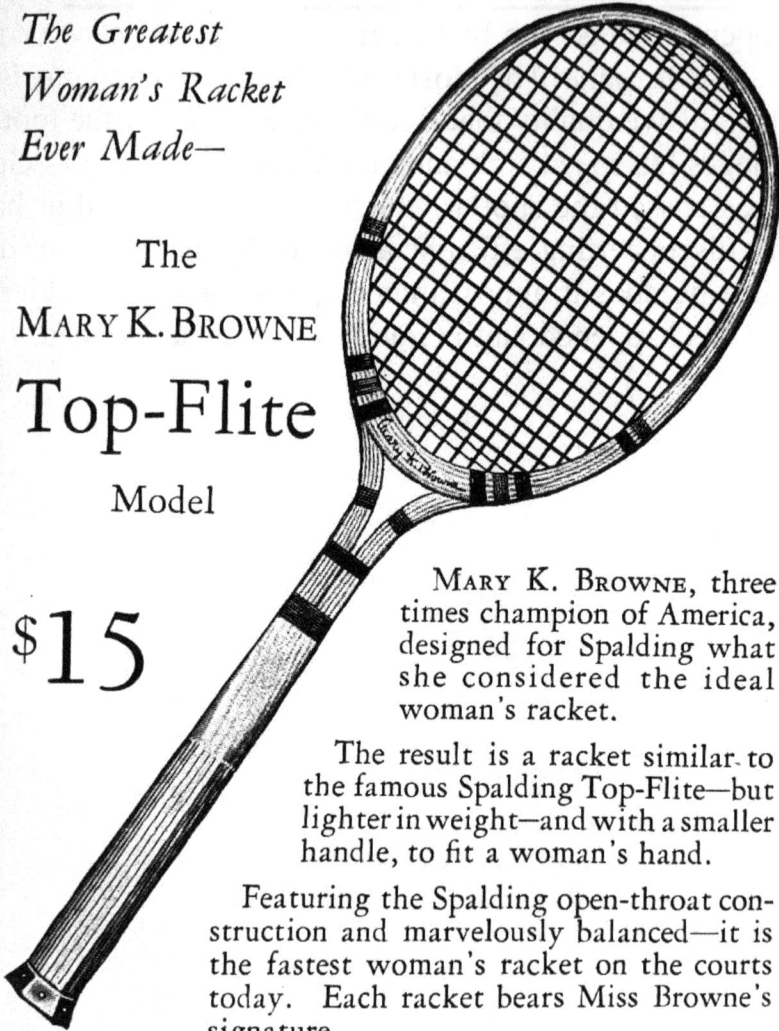

MARY K. BROWNE, three times champion of America, designed for Spalding what she considered the ideal woman's racket.

The result is a racket similar to the famous Spalding Top-Flite—but lighter in weight—and with a smaller handle, to fit a woman's hand.

Featuring the Spalding open-throat construction and marvelously balanced—it is the fastest woman's racket on the courts today. Each racket bears Miss Browne's signature.

Stores in all principal cities

A.G. Spalding & Bros.

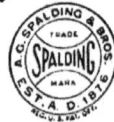

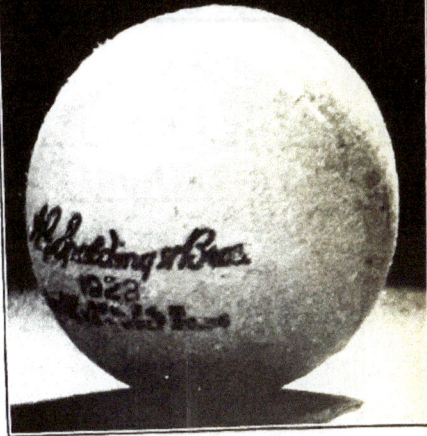

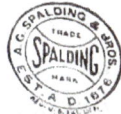

ABOUT THE AUTHORS

"With what little I know, allow me to introduce my co-author, Don DeNevi"

by Kie Foreman

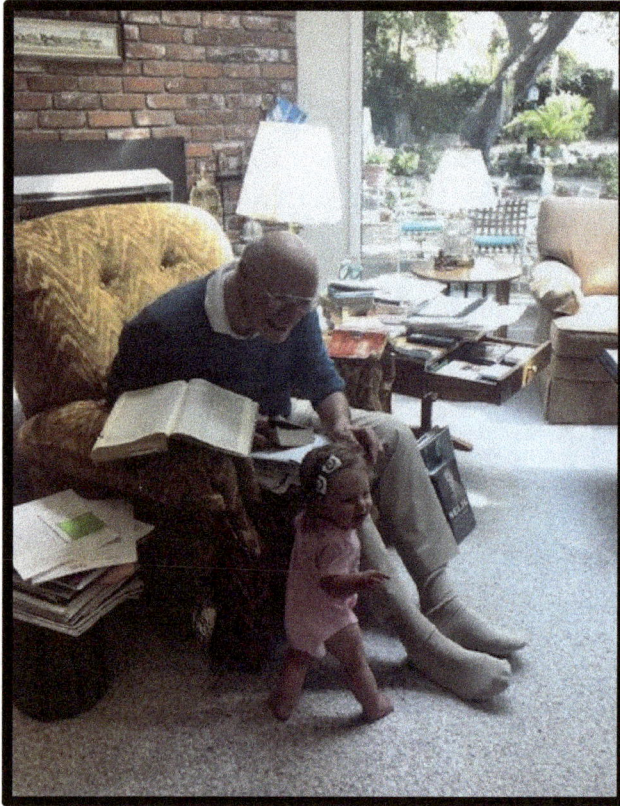

(Juliet, granddaughter of friend Angela, learning to walk is now demanding Don read from Mary K. Browne's "Top Flight Tennis" written and published in 1928. "Brownie" is one of juliet's favorite authors.)

There are so many intricately combined parts of him that he's impossible to define - - high school teacher, counselor, university associate professor, watercolor artist, fiction and nonfiction author, book reviewer for 44 years, and after retirement, prison teacher and Supervisor of Recreation at Soledad, Salinas Valley, and San Quentin State Prison. He joined the Pebble Beach Club membership in 1992, and I've known him since I replaced Tony Trabert's son, Mike, as Director of Tennis of the Beach & Tennis Club in 2000.

Of all my favorite impressions of Don was when at the beginning of our co-authorship in my office, he mentioned in passing while pausing to gaze out the window how during his 69 years on the courts, in his early years twice a week, later in life, four and five times a week, that he consciously and deliberately cheated on three occasions while playing against his closest friends. "I've never forgotten any of the three. I called three balls out that were good in order to beat guys I really loved and respected. I betrayed them. I still remember the expression on each face. What kind of man does that? I'm long past the embarrassed and anger-at-myself stages. "But I've never forgotten how I also betrayed and cheated the integrity of the game. And, for what? I will never forgive myself."

(Kie Foreman)

"O.K., O.K., now that that's over, let's get back to Kie, the real tenniser"

By Don DeNevi

Although his detailed resume as Director of Tennis at the Beach and Tennis Club next door to the Lodge in Pebble Beach, California, reads like a fictitious fable of marvelous mythical tennis court events and happenings, it is Kie's cogent chronicling of his 36-year career, line by line, in professional tennis instruction that's more mesmerizing. Spanning seven single-spaced pages, he proudly lists his responsibilities for all tennis related activities; all aspects of club operations; being held accountable for all club instruction, clinics, tournaments, interclub team competition; U.S.T.A. team rivalries; after school youth classes; summer junior programs; youth, junior, and teenage summer programs; junior exhibition matches; and special instructional teaching during weekends. An avid tenniser can't help but smile and genuflect.

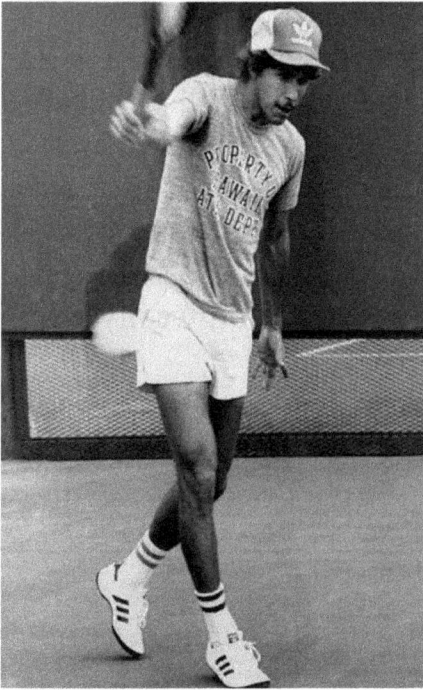

There is little question why Kie's leadership skills, tennis knowledge, and on-court accomplishments, and teaching ability as a tennis coach-instructor impress visiting tennis administrators from similar clubs (none in the world more aesthetically welcoming than Pebble's). Between 2002 and 2020, our club was ranked as one of the top 100 tennis resorts in the world by Tennis Resorts On-Line. Space limits his additional management successes; singles and doubles tournaments won and trophies presented; the almost immediate increases in attendance wherever he was recruited as Director of Tennis, i.e., Head Men's Tennis Coach, Idaho State University; Willow Creek Racquet Club, Eugene, Oregon; Sun Valley Tennis Club,

194

Sun Valley, Idaho; and the Boulder Resort and Club, Scottsdale, Arizona. For the past three plus decades, he has managed the Beach & Tennis Club at the Lodge of Pebble Beach.

There, the top management team, unit staffs, and swim and tennis members (currently, 1,500+) acknowledge him as a charitable legend, as do northern California drive-in tennis weekenders, and week-long visitors from across the country. Yet, such achievements blanche in comparison to who Kie, the man, is. His staunchest admirers claim, as I do, he encompasses chivalry, kindness, gentleness, and positiveness. Recently, on the court next to ours, while my foursome changed sides, I overheard a fine middle-aged single woman-member comment to her fellow three players, "Kie is such a gentleman, all the best ones around here are. But he's special and honorable. And, what a work ethic. His day begins at 8:00am, yet he's here at 7:30am, on the court at 7:45am, with the club vacuum, blowing away all the night's debris. No matter when you arrive to play, the courts are all spotlessly clean, you can eat pancakes off them." When I whispered what was said to my three tennis partners that morning, one simply nodded and said softly, "Women know. It's his kindliness and gentleness that impress them. "Plus, his gracious courteousness and politeness. To us men, it's his absolute loyalty to the game of tennis, and thus to all of us. No one I've ever known has commingled the art of professional instruction, even to two- and three-year-olds, and sincere and dedicated passion for the learner than in his unique personality."

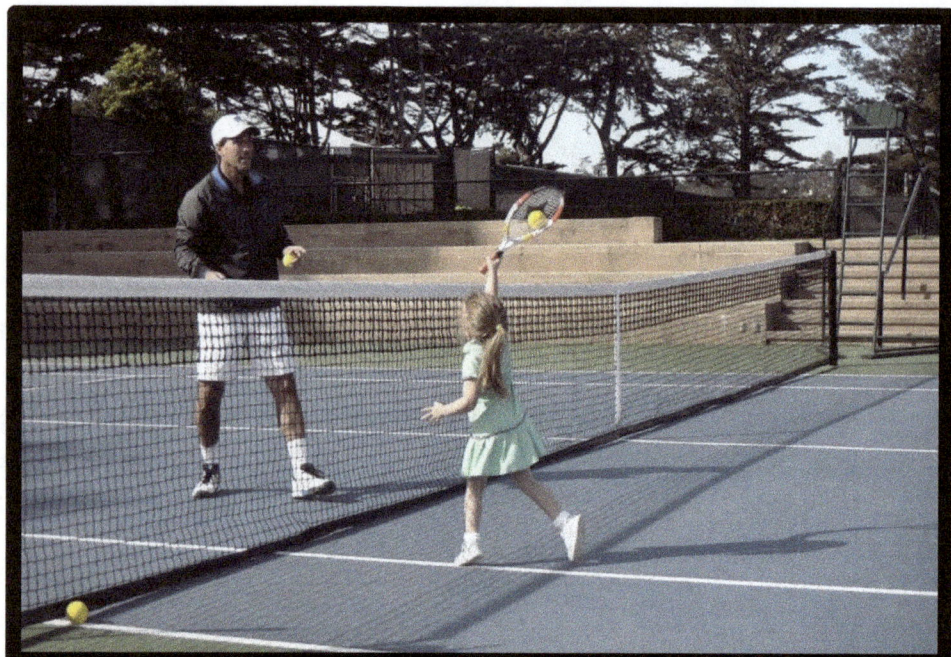

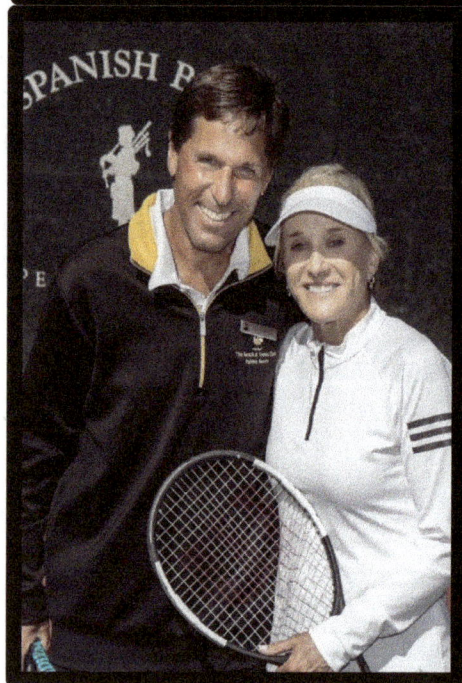

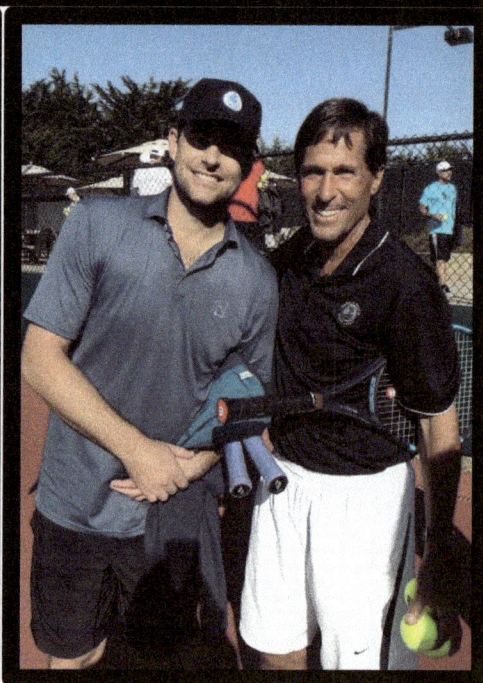

(Kie Foreman with Juliet, Tracy Austin and Andy Roddick)

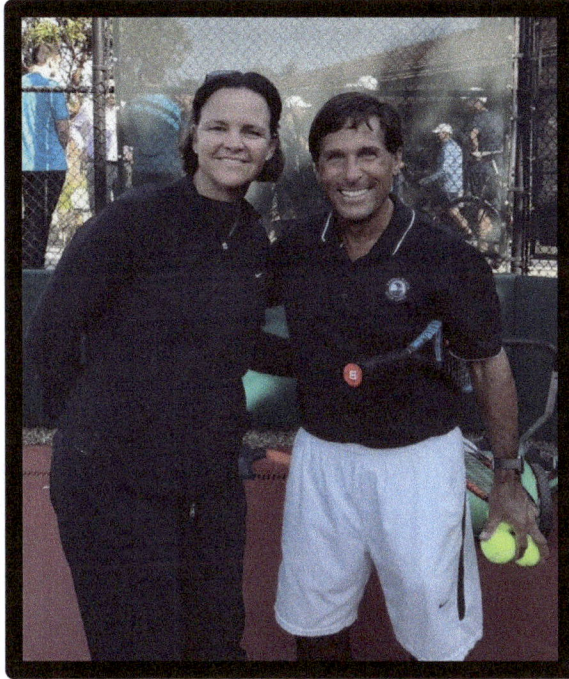

(Kie Foreman and Lindsay Davenport and Brad Gilbert)

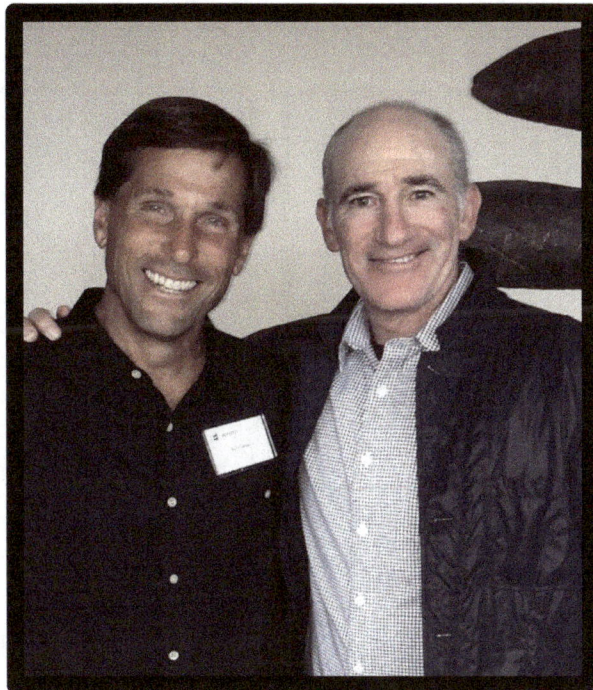

Anna Likes to Play Tennis with Pop Pop, Stewart Frazer

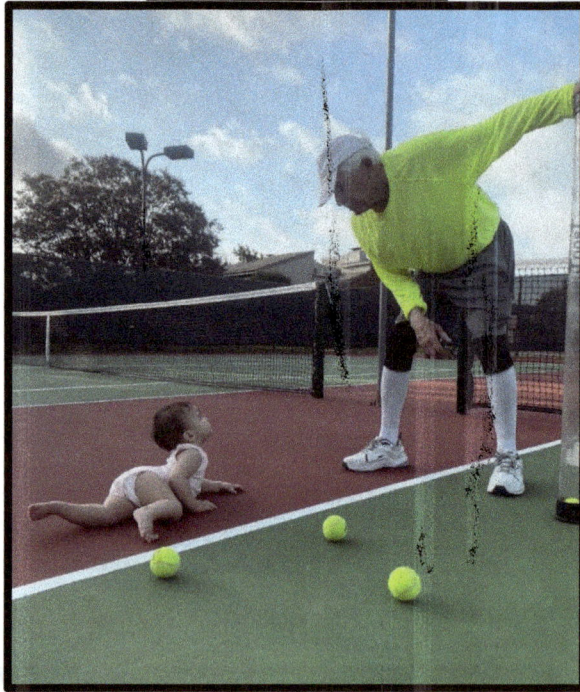

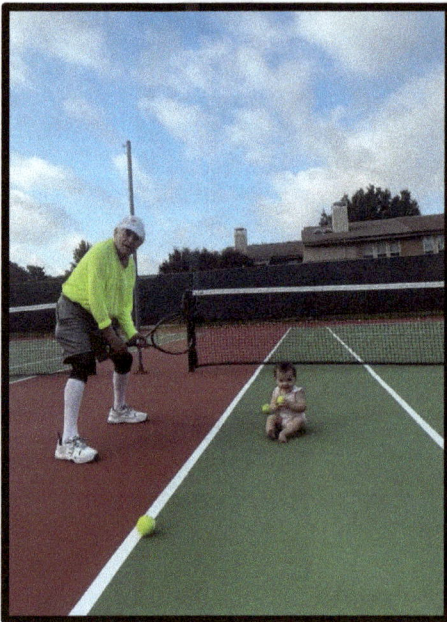

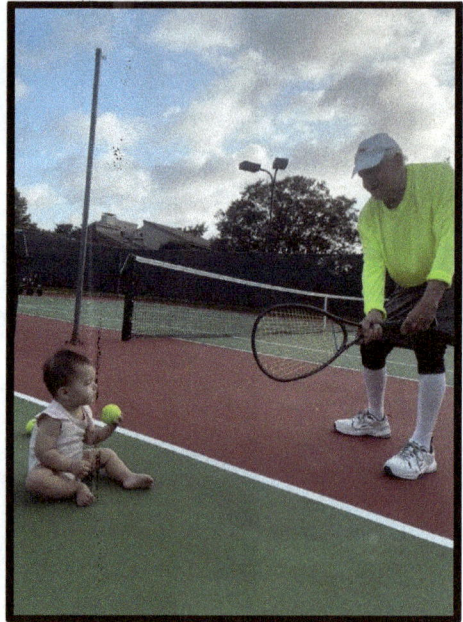

TO THE READER

Why not take a moment to write a letter to Kie and Don, who promise to respond, on how you were introduced to tennis, at what age, and by whom? If you can recall, what were your first impressions, and who lead you on? Describe your later inducements and those personalities, including parents, relatives, and friends who played pivotal roles in your tennis growth and development. You have our word on it, we will answer.

SEND TO:
Kie Foreman, Director of Tennis, Beach & Tennis Club
P.O. Box 1128,
Pebble Beach, CA. 93953
http://www.pebblebeach.com/
foremank@pebblebeach.com

www.ingramcontent.com/pod-product-compliance
Lightning Source LLC
Chambersburg PA
CBHW061753260326

41914CB00006B/1092